The nursing

assistant

in Hematology

MARTIN STERLING

Table of contents

8

« Hematology is where every cell counts, where every gesture heals, and where every day reminds us of the fragility and strength of life. »

Chapter 1

Understanding the Hematology Department

Definition of hematology: what is it?
Introduction to the medical specialty and the main pathologies treated (leukemia, lymphoma, myeloma, etc.).

Hematology is a complex and fascinating medical specialty dedicated to the study of blood, hematopoietic organs (bone marrow, lymph nodes, spleen) and the diseases that affect them. As a discipline, it lies at the crossroads of biology, immunology and oncology, encompassing a broad spectrum of pathologies from benign conditions to particularly aggressive blood cancers.

The main diseases treated in hematology are often grouped under the generic term "hematological malignancies", among which leukemias, lymphomas and myelomas occupy a prominent place. These diseases affect blood cells, blood cell precursors or immune cells, and require specific, often multidisciplinary, treatment.

Leukemias are cancers of the cells of the bone marrow, where blood cells are produced. They are characterized by an uncontrolled proliferation of immature cells, called blasts, which prevent the normal development of red blood cells, white blood cells and platelets. Leukemias are generally classified into two broad categories: acute leukemias, which progress rapidly and require immediate treatment, and chronic leukemias, which progress more slowly but can lead to serious complications if left untreated. In acute myeloid leukemia (AML), for example, immature myeloid cells invade the bone marrow, preventing the production of normal cells. Acute lymphoblastic leukemia (ALL), on the other hand, affects lymphocytes, essential immune cells.

Lymphomas are cancers that affect the lymphatic system, in particular the lymph nodes, spleen and thymus. They are characterized by an uncontrolled proliferation of lymphocytes, the cells that play a crucial role in immune defense. Lymphomas fall into two main categories: Hodgkin's lymphoma, which is relatively rare and often associated with a good prognosis if treated in time, and non-Hodgkin's lymphomas, which include a wide variety of more or less aggressive subtypes. Lymphoma treatment can include chemotherapy, radiotherapy and, in some cases, stem cell transplantation.

Finally, **myeloma** affects plasma cells, a type of white blood cell specialized in antibody production. In multiple myeloma, these cells proliferate uncontrollably in the bone marrow, disrupting the production of other blood cells and leading to complications such as infections, anemia and bone lesions. There is currently no cure for multiple myeloma, but treatments such as chemotherapy, immunomodulating agents and stem cell transplants can control its progression and improve patients' quality of life.

In addition to these three main categories, hematology also encompasses non-malignant diseases such as anemias, coagulation disorders (such as hemophilia) and thrombotic diseases. One of the major challenges of this specialty is that each disease, each patient, has its own particularities that require individualized management. Constantly evolving knowledge in molecular biology and genetics has led to considerable advances in the diagnosis, prognosis and treatment of hematological diseases, paving the way for more targeted and effective therapies.

Hematology is more than just the study of blood disorders. It offers a global perspective on a patient's health, integrating biological, therapeutic and psychological elements, as patient follow-up is often lengthy and requires particular attention to quality of life and support throughout the care process.

Hematology department structure and organization
The different departments (clinical hematology, intensive care units, bone marrow transplantation) and the organization of the care team.

Hematology is a specialty requiring rigorous organization and close collaboration between different departments, each with a very specific role in patient care. These services are generally divided into several distinct units, ranging from clinical hematology to intensive care units and bone marrow transplant services. Each of these care environments has its own particularities, and all are built around a patient-centered approach, with multidisciplinary teams working together to deliver the best possible care.

The **Clinical Hematology Department** is often the main point of entry for patients with hematological pathologies, whether benign or malignant. In this department, symptoms are assessed, diagnostic tests are carried out (blood tests, bone marrow biopsies, imaging examinations) and appropriate treatments are put in place. This may be outpatient or inpatient for patients undergoing chemotherapy, immunotherapy or targeted therapy. The care team, made up of hematologists, nurses, nurses' aides, psychologists and dieticians, work together to adjust treatments as the disease progresses. Caregivers play a key role in patient comfort and supervision, looking after their day-to-day well-being and ensuring smooth communication between the patient and the rest of the care team.

Hematology Intensive Care Units (HICUs) are specialized wards for critically ill patients. These units are particularly important for patients with serious complications related to their treatment or disease, such as severe infections, bleeding or organ failure. Immunosuppressed patients following intensive chemotherapy or bone marrow transplants can be particularly vulnerable, requiring continuous monitoring and highly technical care. Caregivers in these units have an indispensable role to play in monitoring vital parameters, assisting patients with daily gestures and implementing strict asepsis protocols to prevent infections. The emotional burden in these units is often high, but cooperation between all team members - resuscitation doctors, specialist nurses, orderlies - ensures that vital emergencies are dealt with quickly and efficiently.

Bone marrow transplantation is one of the most complex areas of hematology. Bone marrow transplantation, or more precisely hematopoietic stem cell transplantation, is often the only curative option for patients suffering from diseases such as acute leukemia or refractory lymphoma. This extremely delicate process involves preparing the patient with myeloablative treatments (high-dose chemotherapy, sometimes radiotherapy) to destroy the diseased bone marrow and enable the implantation of new stem cells. Post-transplant care is intense, focusing on infection prevention and the management of graft-versus-host syndrome (GVH), a frequent complication where the transplanted cells attack the patient's tissues. Caregivers, alongside specialized nurses, are at the heart of this care, meticulously monitoring symptoms, ensuring the cleanliness and strict hygiene of rooms, and providing essential psychological support to patients often exhausted by the process.

The organization of the care team in these different departments is based on continuous collaboration and fluid communication. Everyone's role is well defined, but it's by working together that we succeed in providing quality care. **Hematology physicians** supervise treatments, establish protocols and ensure precise clinical follow-up of patients. **Nurses**, specialized in hematology, administer treatments, monitor vital signs and manage the side effects of heavy therapies. **Nurses' aides**, meanwhile, ensure the day-to-day well-being of patients, taking charge of hygiene care, observing clinical signs and passing on crucial information to other team members. Their role is often that of first contact with patients, enabling them to detect the slightest signs of discomfort or complications, and to alert quickly if necessary.

Teamwork is fundamental in these departments, and care coordination is based on **regular** staff **meetings**, where all the professionals involved meet to discuss complex cases, adjust treatments and exchange best practices. This organization, based on genuine synergy between all the players involved, enables us to cope with the complexity of hematology care, while always placing the patient at the center of all decisions.

Hematology patients: a specific population

Patient profile: often immunocompromised, at risk of infection and requiring special care.

The profile of patients treated in haematology is unique, due to the nature of the diseases that affect them and the often severe treatments they receive. The majority of these patients, whether suffering from leukemia, lymphoma, myeloma or other hematological pathologies, have one thing in common: a weakened or even severely compromised immune system. This immunodepression, which may be pathological in origin or the result of treatment (chemotherapy, radiotherapy, immunosuppressants), exposes patients to major risks of infection, and calls for heightened vigilance on the part of care teams.

Hematological patients are particularly vulnerable to infection, as their immune systems are often unable to react effectively against pathogens. In leukemia, for example, diseased blood cells gradually replace healthy ones, disrupting the normal production of white blood cells, essential for immune defense. Added to this is the fact that treatments designed to eliminate cancer cells, such as chemotherapy or bone marrow transplants, also destroy residual immune cells. As a result, these patients find themselves temporarily defenseless against bacteria, viruses and even fungi, which can trigger serious or even fatal infections, even from microbes normally harmless to a healthy person.

This immune fragility calls for **special care** that goes beyond standard care. Asepsis protocols are strictly enforced in hematology departments. Patients' rooms, especially those undergoing post-transplant or intensive chemotherapy, are often sterile or laminar-flow rooms, where the air is filtered to limit particles and infectious agents. Every gesture made by nurses, doctors or even visitors must be preceded by rigorous precautions: masks, gloves, gowns and meticulous hand disinfection. On a day-to-day basis, the nursing auxiliary plays a vital role in maintaining this safe environment, ensuring that protocols are strictly adhered to to minimize the risk of infection.

The immunosuppression of haematology patients also calls for appropriate personal care. Particular attention is paid to personal hygiene, as even a small skin lesion, irritation or oral infection can quickly develop into a serious complication. Hygiene care is carried out with extreme delicacy, to avoid irritation or injury. What's more, patients are often very weak and bedridden, and require assistance with the most basic daily tasks, such as washing, feeding and moving around. Caregivers must therefore combine technical skills with human attention to provide care tailored to these specific needs.

In addition to the risk of infection, these patients often present **hemorrhagic complications** due to abnormal platelet production or rapid platelet destruction, leading to an increased risk of bleeding. This phenomenon is common in patients undergoing chemotherapy, as the treatment affects not only malignant cells, but also platelets, essential for blood clotting. Even a simple gesture, such as brushing the teeth or physical mobilization, can cause severe bleeding. This requires rigorous monitoring for signs of bleeding, whether through bruising, bleeding from the nose or gums, or more serious internal bleeding. Caregivers are trained to spot these signs and report them immediately to adjust care or prevent any worsening.

Last but not least, these patients, often faced with long and trying treatments, also have **specific** psychological needs. Hematological pathologies, particularly when they are malignant, are often synonymous with a long medical course, made up of relapses, aggressive treatments and uncertainties. This battle against the disease generates great moral and physical fatigue, associated with anxiety, stress and even depression. The role of caregivers, and in particular orderlies, is central here. As the first point of contact with patients, they are often the first line of psychological support, offering a sympathetic ear, reassurance and a calming presence in a care environment that can be highly technical and dehumanizing. They accompany patients through difficult times, look after their well-being and bring a touch of humanity to a hospital environment sometimes perceived as hostile.

Chapter 2

The key role of the hematology caregiver

Hygiene and comfort care for hematology patients
The importance of daily care to prevent infections in immunocompromised patients.

In immunocompromised patients, as is often the case in haematology, infection prevention is a top priority and relies heavily on the quality of daily care. The weakening of the immune system, whether due to the disease itself or to aggressive treatments such as chemotherapy or bone marrow transplants, makes these patients extremely vulnerable to infection. For these patients, a simple infection, which would be benign in a healthy person, can quickly turn into a serious medical emergency, leading to sepsis or other potentially fatal complications. This is where daily care comes into its own, as it represents one of the main barriers against infectious agents.

Personal hygiene is one of the first lines of defense in preventing infection in immunocompromised patients. This care goes far beyond simple patient comfort; it is essential to reduce the microbial load on the skin and mucous membranes, which are the main entry points for germs into the body. The skin, as the first protective barrier, is particularly vulnerable when immunity is weakened. In bed-ridden or very weak patients, meticulous care is needed to avoid skin infections such as bedsores or dermatitis. This includes daily cleaning, regular changes of dressings and clothing, and constant monitoring of high-risk areas, such as skin folds, catheter sites or areas where the skin is in prolonged contact with sheets or the chair.

Particular attention to oral hygiene is also crucial. In immunocompromised patients, the mouth is a particularly sensitive area. Treatments such as chemotherapy or radiotherapy can cause mucositis, painful inflammation of the mucous membranes, which not only makes eating difficult, but also exposes the patient to an increased risk of fungal or bacterial infections. Daily care therefore consists of gentle brushing, often accompanied by antiseptic mouthwashes to limit germ proliferation. This gesture, which may seem simple, plays a fundamental role in preventing oral infections, which can easily spread throughout the body and lead to serious complications.

The patient's environment must also be carefully maintained. Every day, orderlies ensure that the patient's room is kept impeccably clean. In haematology departments, and particularly in units caring for patients with bone marrow aplasia (a period when the bone marrow no longer produces blood cells), strict measures are put in place to minimize the presence of germs. This involves not only rigorous surface cleaning, but also the use of devices such as laminar flow chambers, which filter the air to prevent the circulation of particles and infectious agents. Nurses are responsible for strict compliance with asepsis protocols, from wearing gloves, masks and gowns to systematic hand disinfection before and after each treatment. These gestures, repeated throughout the day, minimize the risk of introducing germs into the patient's environment, creating a protective bubble around him/her.

Daily care also includes careful monitoring of invasive devices, such as central venous catheters, peripheral lines or implantable chambers, often used to administer treatments or infusions. These devices, essential for treating hematological patients, are also potential entry points for infections if not properly maintained. The nursing auxiliary therefore ensures the daily cleanliness of these devices, by applying sterile dressings and monitoring for signs of redness, inflammation or exudation around the insertion sites. Any abnormality detected is immediately reported to the medical team, to prevent any local infection that could rapidly spread if not promptly treated.

It is also essential to remember that diet is an integral part of daily care to prevent infection. Immunocompromised patients often need to follow specific diets, as certain foods may contain pathogens that can cause foodborne infections. For example, raw fruit and vegetables, unpasteurized or undercooked products are often forbidden. The caregiver plays a key role here, ensuring that meals comply with strict dietary guidelines and helping the patient to eat correctly, as good nutrition is essential to support the body weakened by treatment.

Finally, beyond technical care, the relational aspect of daily care also contributes to infection prevention. Immunocompromised patients are often very isolated, both physically and emotionally, due to strict isolation measures. This loneliness can lead to low morale and even depression, which in turn can further weaken the body. The caregiver's daily presence, attentiveness and interaction contribute not only to the patient's mental well-being, but also indirectly to the body's resilience to infection. A psychologically-supported patient is better able to follow care instructions scrupulously and to remain active as much as possible, thus contributing to his or her recovery.

Monitoring vital signs and clinical observation
Close monitoring of vital signs and clinical manifestations (fever, signs of infection, bleeding).

Close monitoring of vital signs and clinical manifestations is a fundamental pillar in the management of haematology patients, particularly those who are immunocompromised or undergoing intensive treatment. These patients, whose state of health can deteriorate rapidly, require heightened vigilance, as slight changes in vital signs or the appearance of subtle symptoms can be a harbinger of serious complications such as infection or haemorrhage. This rigorous monitoring, often carried out by care assistants in close collaboration with the nursing and medical teams, is crucial to identifying emergency situations early and responding appropriately.

One of the most important vital signs to monitor in hematology is **body temperature**. In an immunocompromised patient, the onset of even a mild fever can be a sign of serious infection, particularly as their weakened immune system is unable to mount an effective response against pathogens. A body temperature above 38°C is considered a potentially serious indicator in this context. However, the absence of fever does not always mean the absence of infection, as some immunocompromised patients may not present with a fever due to their inability to develop an adequate inflammatory response. This is why regular temperature monitoring, combined with ongoing assessment of the patient's general condition, is essential. Undetected fever or untreated infection can rapidly progress to sepsis, a potentially fatal complication. In this context, the nursing auxiliary plays a vital role by regularly taking the patient's temperature, detecting temperature rises and immediately reporting any abnormalities to the medical team.

Monitoring **heart rate** and **blood pressure** is also crucial. Tachycardia (increased heart rate) or hypotension (falling blood pressure) can be early indicators of complications, such as septic shock or hemorrhage. A patient with a significant drop in blood pressure may be bleeding internally, particularly if the patient is on anticoagulant therapy or in bone marrow failure, a period when platelet counts are drastically reduced, increasing the risk of bleeding. Caregivers, by regularly taking blood pressure and monitoring pulse, are in the front line in spotting these warning signs. Persistent tachycardia or a drop in blood pressure, even if there are no other apparent symptoms, must be reported without delay, to enable prompt treatment.

Signs of infection go beyond simple temperature monitoring. An immunocompromised patient may show signs of infection through subtle alterations in general condition: increased fatigue, confusion, restlessness or chills may be early indicators. Infections can also manifest themselves locally, as in the case of catheters, where redness, pain, purulent discharge or tenderness around the insertion site should be closely monitored. Urinary tract infections are also common in these patients, and signs such as abdominal pain, painful urination or cloudy urine should alert caregivers. Finally, pulmonary infections, such as pneumonia, are of particular concern, and can manifest themselves as coughing, breathing difficulties, or low oxygen saturation. Here again, caregivers play an essential role, as they are often the first to observe these subtle changes in the patient's behavior or clinical condition, enabling them to act quickly in collaboration with the medical team.

In addition to signs of infection, monitoring for **signs of hemorrhage** is essential in hematology patients. Thrombocytopenia, a low platelet count, is a frequent complication in these patients, particularly those in bone marrow aplasia or receiving myelotoxic treatments. A low platelet count increases the risk of bleeding, both externally and internally. Caregivers must be particularly vigilant for spontaneous bruising, bleeding gums during oral or dental care, or blood in urine or stools. Nasal bleeding or a large hematoma may seem minor, but in a thrombocytopenic patient, these manifestations may be the sign of a generalized hemorrhagic tendency requiring platelet transfusion or emergency medical intervention.

In the case of **internal bleeding**, the signs may be more subtle and difficult to detect. Sudden pallor, an increase in heart rate, a drop in blood pressure, or abdominal pain may be indicators of gastrointestinal hemorrhage or another form of internal bleeding. This is why constant monitoring of vital signs, combined with careful clinical assessment, is essential. The caregiver, by being present with the patient on a daily basis, is often the one who picks up these weak signals and enables rapid intervention.

The importance of this close monitoring lies not only in taking vital signs, but also in the ability to observe and interpret sometimes subtle, but potentially critical, clinical signs. Through their close contact with patients, orderlies develop an ability to detect changes in patient behavior or appearance that may signal the onset of infection, bleeding or other complications. They play a central role in the vigilance system set up around hematology patients, enabling them to react rapidly to any deterioration in the patient's condition.

Pain and comfort management in collaboration with the nursing team
The caregiver's role in assessing the patient's pain and discomfort, and in administering non-drug treatments.

The caregiver's role in assessing pain and discomfort in hematology patients is essential, as these patients, often faced with heavy treatments and serious pathologies, regularly live with a variety of physical pains and discomforts. Pain can be acute or chronic, caused by the disease itself or by its treatment, and accurate assessment is crucial to providing appropriate care. Because of their daily proximity to the patient, caregivers are often the first to observe signs of pain, even when it is not expressed verbally. This gives them a key role in detecting suffering, adapting care and administering non-drug treatments to relieve the patient.

Pain assessment relies above all on observation and careful listening. In haematology, patients may experience pain of various kinds: bone pain linked to metastases or myeloma, joint pain, neuropathic pain after chemotherapy, or visceral pain after bone marrow transplants. Some patients express their pain clearly, but others, particularly when exhausted or undergoing heavy treatment, may find it difficult to verbalize it. The caregiver therefore plays a fundamental role in listening for non-verbal signals: pain mimics, agitation, rapid breathing, rigid posture or moaning may be signs that the patient is in pain. He or she must be able to spot these signs, however discreet, and report them to the nursing and medical team, enabling rapid adaptation of care or analgesic treatment.

Dialogue with the patient is also an essential part of this assessment. The caregiver, through his or her regular presence and trusting relationship with the patient, is often in the front line of gathering the latter's feelings about his or her pain. They can ask patients about the intensity, location and type of pain they feel. This communication helps us to target our interventions more effectively, as each type of pain requires a different response. For example, neuropathic pain may require specific treatment or adapted physical interventions. In some cases, the discomfort may be more diffuse, linked to prolonged positioning, aches and pains, or generalized weakness induced by treatment. These discomforts, though often underestimated, can severely impair the patient's quality of life if not managed proactively.

In this context, the caregiver plays a crucial role in the administration of **non-drug treatments**, which can provide significant relief in addition to medication. These non-pharmacological treatments, often based on physical care, relaxation or comfort techniques, are particularly valuable in hematology, where pain and discomfort can be constant and difficult to relieve with medication alone.

One of the key aspects of non-drug care is **mobilization and physical rehabilitation**. Hematology patients, who are often bedridden or severely weakened by treatment, regularly suffer from pain associated with immobility: muscular pain, joint pain or pain associated with the formation of bedsores. The caregiver, in collaboration with the physiotherapist, ensures that the patient is regularly mobilized, according to his or her abilities, to avoid these discomforts. This may include regular position changes, passive mobilization exercises, or the installation of positioning cushions to relieve certain areas of the body. These interventions help prevent the pain associated with prolonged immobilization, and promote the patient's overall comfort.

At the same time, the caregiver can suggest **relaxation techniques** or comfort treatments to reduce the sensation of pain. Simple gestures such as light massage of painful areas, gentle hygiene care to avoid irritation, or the application of cold or hot compresses can all help to improve patient comfort. Although non-invasive, these techniques often bring significant relief, especially for patients suffering from chronic or residual pain after treatment. Massages, in particular, release muscular tension and provide a moment of physical and psychological comfort.

Guided relaxation, **controlled breathing** or the use of **positive visualization** techniques are other methods that can be suggested to patients in pain. These simple but effective techniques help to reduce the perception of pain by diverting attention and promoting a state of mental calm. The caregiver, by virtue of his or her proximity and ability to listen, is well placed to propose these approaches at times when the patient feels overwhelmed by pain or anxiety. These interventions, although non-medical, help to improve the patient's emotional state, which plays a crucial role in overall pain management.

Another important aspect of the caregiver's role is the creation of a **soothing environment**. Patient comfort depends not only on direct care, but also on the atmosphere in which the patient is treated. Ensuring that the room is clean, quiet and well-lit, and that the patient has access to everything he or she needs (water, personal items, entertainment) contributes to his or her general well-being and can help reduce discomfort. Attention to these small details can make the hospital experience less stressful and more bearable, which is essential for patients who are often hospitalized for long periods.

Finally, the nursing auxiliary acts as a **mediator** between the patient and the nursing team. By carefully observing the evolution of pain or discomfort, they can quickly signal any changes in the patient's condition, enabling them to adapt their pain medication or care. This communication is crucial, as it prevents pain from becoming entrenched or worsening, thereby improving the patient's quality of life.

Psychological support for patients and their families

Listening and emotional support in the often stressful context of hematology.

Listening and emotional support are central to the day-to-day work in hematology, a specialty where patients are not only confronted with serious, often disabling illnesses, but also with long and demanding treatments. This medical context is particularly difficult for patients, who have to cope not only with physical pain and treatment-related side-effects, but also with profound anxiety linked to the seriousness of their illness and uncertainties as to how their state of health will evolve. It is in this context that the nursing auxiliary, in addition to its technical skills, plays a crucial role in providing patients with attentive listening and constant emotional support.

Emotional support often begins with the ability to simply be there for the patient, to establish a relationship of trust based on listening, caring and availability. For many hematology patients, the hospital becomes a familiar place, where they spend long periods due to intensive treatments such as chemotherapy, bone marrow transplants or post-transplant care. Because of their proximity to patients, orderlies are often one of their most regular contacts, accompanying them on a daily basis in moments of weakness, doubt or pain. In this way, they become an important point of reference in a medical environment that is sometimes perceived as hostile or frightening.

Listening, in this context, goes beyond simply hearing what the patient says. It involves **active listening**, i.e. paying close attention not only to the patient's words, but also to his or her silences, bodily expressions and general state of mind. Patients with haematological diseases are often overwhelmed by complex emotions: fear of death, frustration with physical limitations, worries about the future or feelings of isolation. By listening, the caregiver enables the patient to verbalize these emotions, to put into words what he or she is feeling, and thus to find some relief from the accumulated anguish. It's not uncommon for patients to confide in the caregiver concerns they don't dare express to their family or even their doctor, for fear of worrying them. This is why listening must be respectful, empathetic and non-judgmental, providing a safe space for patients to express their emotions.

When it comes to emotional care, **psychological support** also takes the form of small, everyday gestures which, although seemingly simple, have a big impact on patients' morale. Whether it's staying a few extra minutes at the bedside of an anxious patient, holding their hand, talking to them to reassure them before a painful treatment, or simply asking them how they really feel, these moments of exchange help to humanize care and bring comfort to days often punctuated by medical protocols. These interactions remind patients that they are not reduced to their illness or symptoms, but that they are first and foremost individuals, whose emotions and psychological needs are just as important as their physical ones.

The **emotional support** offered by the caregiver also extends to the patient's family, who are themselves often in great distress in the face of their loved one's illness. Family members, although present and eager to help, may feel powerless or helpless in the face of the seriousness of the situation. The caregiver can play a mediating role by explaining care, answering practical questions or providing moral support to exhausted relatives. The caregiver helps them to better understand what the patient is going through, and gives them the tools they need to better support the patient. This help is invaluable, as it enables families to feel more involved in the care process and less isolated in the face of worry.

It is also important to note that emotional support in haematology is not limited to the acute phase of a patient's illness. It also extends to periods of remission, which, although marked by a degree of relief, can also give rise to fears of recurrence. The caregiver is often on hand to allay these anxieties, offering a comforting ear and encouraging words. What's more, as the disease progresses or treatment fails, patient support becomes even more crucial. The caregiver then intervenes not only to relieve physical pain, but also to offer essential psychological support in moments of deep despair or sadness.

Finally, in cases where treatments are no longer curative and the patient enters a palliative phase, the caregiver becomes a **pillar of end-of-life support**. In this particularly delicate situation, the role of emotional support takes on an even deeper dimension. Patients, often confronted with the idea of death, need a reassuring presence, able to listen without judging, and to accompany them in their final moments with respect and dignity. The caregiver, in this context, ensures that the patient feels surrounded, that he is not left alone to face his fears, and that he retains some control over his last days, respecting his wishes and ensuring his comfort. Emotional support also extends to the patient's loved ones, who also need to be accompanied in their impending bereavement.

Chapter 3

Specific hematology procedures and techniques

Strict asepsis protocols in hematology

The importance of protective isolation measures and rigorous disinfection techniques to limit infectious risks.

In hematology, patients are particularly vulnerable to infection due to their immunosuppression, often induced by the disease itself or by the aggressive treatments they receive, such as chemotherapy, radiotherapy or bone marrow transplants. These treatments severely affect immune cell production, leaving patients defenseless against pathogens. In this context, infection prevention becomes an absolute priority to ensure their safety and recovery. One of the most effective strategies for protecting these patients is protective isolation, accompanied by rigorous disinfection techniques.

Protective isolation is an essential measure for limiting the exposure of immunocompromised patients to infectious agents present in the hospital environment or carried by those around them. Because of their immune fragility, these patients can develop serious infections from bacteria, viruses or fungi that are normally harmless to healthy people. Isolation aims to create a barrier between the patient and these pathogens, reducing as far as possible the risk of exogenous infection. Isolation rooms, often equipped with laminar flow air filtration systems, provide a controlled environment where particles and germs are continuously filtered. This minimizes the risks associated with ambient air, particularly for patients in bone marrow aplasia, a period when their bodies produce virtually no blood cells, including defense cells.

In these rooms, every entry and exit is meticulously supervised. Caregivers, visitors and even medical staff must follow strict protocols to avoid introducing outside microbes. This includes the wearing of masks, gloves, gowns, and sometimes even caps or shoe covers, to limit the risk of contamination through direct contact or by air. On a daily basis, orderlies ensure that these measures are respected in all circumstances, and play an active role in implementing and maintaining these protocols. They are often the first to remind patients of the importance of these measures, and to ensure that all the necessary equipment is available at the entrance to the room. Their role is crucial, as a single oversight can expose the patient to a major infectious risk.

Rigorous disinfection of surfaces, medical devices and hands is also an integral part of these isolation measures. Immunocompromised patients are particularly susceptible to nosocomial infections, which can be transmitted by simple contact with contaminated surfaces or non-sterile instruments. Nurses and orderlies must therefore comply with strict asepsis rules. Every gesture must be preceded by meticulous hand disinfection, using a hydroalcoholic solution or soap and water according to current protocols. This includes not only washing hands before and after every patient contact, but also after handling any object or equipment in the patient's environment.

Medical devices, such as central venous catheters, peripheral lines or implantable chambers, are also potential entry points for infections. Maintaining these devices requires absolute rigor in terms of asepsis. Every manipulation must be carried out under sterile conditions, with regular dressing changes and continuous monitoring for signs of infection, such as redness, swelling or purulent discharge around insertion sites. The nursing auxiliary, as a local professional, plays a key role in this daily monitoring, quickly spotting warning signs and alerting the nursing or medical team if necessary.

Cleaning surfaces in the patient's room is another essential aspect of infection prevention. Everything in contact with the patient or his or her immediate environment must be regularly disinfected: door handles, alarm buttons, remote controls, furniture, etc. These surfaces, often handled by the patient or nursing staff, can become vectors of transmission if not disinfected. These surfaces, often handled by the patient or nursing staff, can become vectors of transmission if they are not disinfected regularly and rigorously. Caregivers therefore ensure that these cleaning protocols are scrupulously respected throughout the day. This also includes frequent changes of bedding and clothing, especially if the patient is sweating, bleeding or discharging.

In addition to these technical measures, the vigilance of nursing staff is constantly called upon to identify signs of infection as soon as they appear. Even in a protected environment, patients can develop internal or opportunistic infections, often linked to their own microbial flora. These infections can manifest themselves as fever, chills, tachycardia, localized pain or more discreet signs, such as a change in general condition. Because of their daily proximity to the patient, caregivers are often the first to observe these symptoms and report them to the medical team, enabling rapid intervention. An infection detected early can be managed rapidly with antibiotics, antivirals or antifungals, while a delay in detection can lead to serious complications, such as sepsis.

It's also important to mention that disinfection and protective isolation don't just apply to the hospital environment. Caregivers play a crucial role in educating patients and their families about good hygiene practices at home, especially for those leaving hospital after a transplant or intensive chemotherapy. They advise on the steps to take to minimize the risk of infection: frequent hand-washing, wearing a mask in public, limiting contact with sick people, and food precautions (avoiding raw or undercooked foods). This education is essential to ensure continuity of protective measures once the patient returns home.

Handling and maintenance of central venous catheters (CVCs), peripheral venous lines and implantable chambers
The caregiver's responsibilities in the care and monitoring of these devices.

Nurses play a central role in the care and monitoring of medical devices used in hematology, including central venous catheters, peripheral lines and implantable chambers. These devices are essential for the administration of treatments such as chemotherapy or blood transfusions, but they also represent potential entry points for infections. Given the heightened vulnerability of immunocompromised patients, the management of these devices demands absolute rigor and constant vigilance. The caregiver, through his or her daily proximity to the patient, is directly involved in the maintenance, observation and prevention of complications linked to these devices.

One of the caregiver's first responsibilities is to ensure **asepsis** during routine care around these devices. Asepsis is crucial to avoid contamination of insertion sites, as an infection introduced via a catheter or implantable chamber can rapidly spread throughout the body, leading to serious complications such as sepsis. This implies strict disinfection procedures before handling the device, whether to change a dressing, reposition a tube or clean the insertion site. Caregivers must systematically use sterile equipment, disinfect their hands with a hydroalcoholic solution and wear sterile gloves before touching the devices. They must also ensure that all materials used for care (compresses, disinfectants, dressings) comply with the department's hygiene protocols.

The **care of central venous catheters** is a particularly delicate task, as these devices are inserted deep into the body and provide a direct route to the bloodstream. Hematology patients, often undergoing chemotherapy or immunosuppressive therapy, are extremely susceptible to infection from these catheters. The caregiver is responsible for keeping the insertion site clean and dry, taking care to change dressings regularly, following strict disinfection protocols. Each dressing change must be carried out with extreme care to avoid moving or contaminating the catheter. In addition, the caregiver must check the condition of the insertion site every day for signs of infection, such as redness, swelling, pain or discharge. If any of these signs appear, they should immediately alert the nursing or medical team for rapid assessment and early management.

Monitoring devices, whether a central line or an implantable chamber, is also an integral part of the caregiver's role. Monitoring goes beyond simple visual observation of the insertion site. He or she must be alert to any sign of malfunction or complication, such as catheter obstruction, extravasation (leakage of fluid into surrounding tissue), or unusual pain reported by the patient. For example, if a patient complains of chest pain or breathing difficulties after using a central venous catheter, this may indicate an embolism or displacement of the device, requiring immediate medical intervention. The caregiver, by being alert to these complaints or symptoms, plays a key role in the early detection of these complications.

Another important aspect of device management is **thrombosis prevention**. Patients with central venous catheters or implantable chambers are at increased risk of blood clots forming at the site of the device, which can lead to serious complications such as pulmonary embolism. The caregiver must be alert to any pain, redness or swelling of the arm or chest on the side where the catheter is placed, which could indicate thrombosis. In addition to this clinical monitoring, he or she is often involved in the regular mobilization of patients, as prolonged immobility can encourage the formation of clots. Mobilization stimulates blood circulation, thereby reducing this risk.

The **relationship with the patient** in managing these devices is also essential. The caregiver must inform and educate the patient on the importance of caring for these devices, in particular by avoiding touching the catheter or insertion site without disinfecting his/her hands, or by reporting any signs of discomfort or infection. This education is particularly important when the patient has to return home with a catheter or an implantable chamber, as he or she will then have to provide part of the care or monitoring himself or herself. The caregiver plays the role of teacher, explaining to the patient how to care for his or her device, what precautions to take, and what signs should alert him or her to seek prompt medical attention.

Finally, the **management of transfusions** and infusions via these devices requires special attention. Hematology patients frequently require infusions of blood products (platelets, red blood cells), chemotherapy or other drugs. The caregiver must ensure that infusions are correctly connected, and monitor their administration to avoid any leaks or complications. They must also regularly check that the catheter or peripheral line is not blocked, and that the flow rate is correct. Constant vigilance is essential to avoid the risk of medication errors or complications linked to incorrect infusion.

Taking samples and caring for patients undergoing chemotherapy
Precautions and support for patients undergoing chemotherapy.

Chemotherapy is one of the most common and effective treatments for patients with hematological cancers, such as leukemia, lymphoma or myeloma. However, due to its mode of action, which targets not only cancer cells but also rapidly dividing healthy cells, chemotherapy is associated with numerous side effects. For this reason, accompanying patients undergoing chemotherapy, and taking specific precautions, are essential to minimize risks and improve patients' quality of life during this trying period. Caregivers play a central role in this process, ensuring close monitoring of side effects, providing moral support and actively contributing to the prevention of complications.

One of the first precautions to be taken is to manage the **risk of infection**, as chemotherapy profoundly weakens the immune system by reducing the production of white blood cells, leaving patients vulnerable to infection. The caregiver must ensure that a strictly aseptic environment is maintained around the patient. This includes rigorous attention to hygiene protocols, including frequent hand washing, surface disinfection and the use of gloves and masks during care. Monitoring for signs of infection, such as fever, chills, or the appearance of redness or pain around medical devices (such as catheters), is also part of the caregiver's daily responsibilities. Any sign of infection should be reported immediately, as even a minor infection can quickly become serious in a patient undergoing chemotherapy.

In addition to the risk of infection, **nausea and vomiting** are very frequent side effects of chemotherapy. Although these symptoms can be partially controlled by antiemetic drugs, they can lead to dehydration and general weakness. The caregiver must ensure that the patient is well hydrated, and encourage light, fractionated feeding to avoid aggravating nausea. They can also suggest non-medicinal techniques to help the patient manage these symptoms, such as relaxation or the use of cold compresses. Monitoring hydration is crucial, as severe dehydration can quickly occur as a result of repeated vomiting, necessitating intravenous rehydration.

Monitoring vital signs is also essential for patients undergoing chemotherapy. Chemotherapy can affect cardiac function, causing variations in blood pressure, heart rate or breathing difficulties. The caregiver, in collaboration with the nursing team, must regularly monitor vital signs to detect any abnormalities and act accordingly. Careful monitoring can prevent or detect serious complications at an early stage, such as cardiotoxicity linked to certain chemotherapeutic agents.

Pain management is one of the major challenges for patients undergoing chemotherapy, as this treatment can lead to diffuse pain, neuropathic pain or bone pain, depending on the substances used and the body's reaction. The caregiver plays a key role in the daily assessment of pain, questioning the patient about his or her feelings and observing non-verbal signs of suffering. They can also provide relief through non-medicinal techniques, such as light massage, position changes or the use of comfort cushions to reduce pressure points. In addition, he/she ensures that prescribed analgesic treatments are correctly administered and effective, promptly reporting any ineffectiveness or worsening of pain to the care team.

Another fundamental aspect of support for patients undergoing chemotherapy is the management of **oral problems**, such as mucositis, an inflammation of the mucous membranes of the mouth that is very common in these patients. Mucositis can make eating painful, complicate hydration and encourage infection. The caregiver must ensure that the patient adopts good oral hygiene, offering gentle antiseptic mouthwashes and making sure that the mouth is well hydrated. It is also important to adapt the patient's diet to avoid any irritating or acidic foods that could aggravate the situation.

Alongside physical care, **psychological and emotional** support for patients undergoing chemotherapy is essential. This treatment is not only physically exhausting, but also psychologically difficult to bear. Patients may experience great fatigue, anxiety, changes in body image (due to hair loss, for example) and emotional distress linked to the uncertainty of the treatment. The caregiver, through regular contact with the patient, can offer invaluable moral support by being a good listener, encouraging the patient to express fears and doubts, and providing comfort at difficult times. This relationship of trust helps to alleviate the isolation felt by patients, and helps them to cope with the psychological challenges imposed by treatment.

In addition, it is important for the caregiver to help **educate the patient** about his or her treatment and the precautions to be taken. This can include advice on managing side effects, precautions to take to avoid infections in the home, and how to adapt daily activities to energy levels. Good information enables patients to better understand what they are going through and to take an active part in their care, which can reduce anxiety and reinforce a sense of control over the disease.

Finally, caring for patients undergoing chemotherapy requires a **multi-disciplinary** approach, where the caregiver works closely with nurses, doctors, psychologists, dieticians and other healthcare professionals. This coordination ensures that every aspect of the patient's well-being is taken into account, from physical symptom management to emotional support and nutritional needs.

Bone marrow post-transplant care
Patient-specific care after transplantation, including management of side effects.

The care of patients after bone marrow transplants, also known as hematopoietic stem cell transplants, is particularly complex and requires rigorous attention due to the many medical and physiological challenges these patients face. After a transplant, patients are often in a highly vulnerable state, both immunologically and physically, and managing side effects becomes a crucial issue. Caregivers play a central role in this comprehensive care, providing close, personalized follow-up to prevent complications, support patients in their convalescence and improve their quality of life.

One of the most important aspects of post-transplant care is **rigorous monitoring of immunosuppression**. After a transplant, the patient's immune system is considerably weakened due to the intensive treatments (chemotherapy or radiotherapy) received prior to transplantation, and the fact that the new transplanted cells take time to reconstitute themselves and regain their immune function. During this period, the risk of infection is extremely high. Patients are often placed in protective isolation to limit their exposure to pathogens. In this context, the nursing auxiliary must ensure that all aseptic measures are scrupulously respected: wearing gloves and masks, disinfecting surfaces and washing hands frequently. He or she must also ensure that all nursing staff and visitors comply with these protocols to protect the patient.

In addition to these isolation precautions, the caregiver must closely monitor for **signs of infection**, as even a minor infection can rapidly escalate in an immunocompromised patient. Regular temperature checks, observation of catheter or venous line insertion sites, and assessment of clinical signs such as fever, chills, cough or localized pain are all part of daily care. Any suspicion of infection should be immediately reported to the medical team for prompt intervention, as untreated infection can lead to serious complications, such as sepsis.

Alongside infectious risks, another major side-effect of transplantation is **graft-versus-host syndrome** (GVH), a frequent and dreaded complication. GVH occurs when the immune cells of the donor (the graft) attack the cells of the recipient (the host), which are considered foreign. The syndrome can be acute or chronic, affecting various organs such as the skin, liver and digestive tract. The caregiver plays a vital role in the early detection of signs of GVH, by daily monitoring of the skin (for redness, rash or itching), stools (for severe diarrhea), and the patient's general condition (loss of appetite, abdominal pain, yellowing of the skin). He is also responsible for ensuring that treatments prescribed to prevent or alleviate GVH, such as immunosuppressants, are correctly administered.

Gastrointestinal side effects are also common after transplantation, particularly in patients suffering from GVH. Diarrhea, nausea, vomiting and abdominal pain are common symptoms, and can have a significant impact on the patient's quality of life and nutritional status. The caregiver must ensure that the patient remains well hydrated and monitor fluid balance, as significant fluid losses due to diarrhea or vomiting can rapidly lead to dehydration. They can also help patients adapt their diet to their digestive tolerance, offering light, easily digestible meals, while monitoring nutritional intake to prevent undernutrition.

Monitoring liver function and signs of liver damage are also essential, as the liver can be a target for GVH. The caregiver should watch for symptoms such as jaundice (yellowing of the skin and eyes), itching, excessive fatigue and changes in stool or urine color. These signs must be reported without delay to enable prompt management, as untreated liver damage can become very serious.

Transplant-related **hematological complications**, such as anemia, thrombocytopenia (low platelets) or neutropenia (low white blood cells), are also common. Caregivers must be particularly vigilant for signs of bleeding in thrombocytopenic patients, such as nosebleeds, bruising or bleeding gums. Similarly, monitoring for signs of anemia, such as pallor, intense fatigue or dizziness, is essential to adapt care and anticipate possible blood transfusions or other medical interventions.

Alongside physical care, **psychological and emotional** support for post-transplant patients is crucial. After a transplant, patients can experience great emotional and moral fatigue, due to prolonged isolation, uncertainties about the success of the transplant, or the multiple side effects they have to cope with. By being close to the patient, the caregiver can offer an attentive and empathetic ear, enabling the patient to express his or her fears, doubts and anxieties. This support is all the more important as the recovery process after a transplant is often long and full of difficult moments. The caregiver can also help the patient maintain a link with loved ones, facilitating communication or visits while respecting isolation protocols.

Finally, it is essential to remember that post-transplant care is part of a **multidisciplinary approach**. Caregivers work closely with nurses, doctors, psychologists, dieticians and physiotherapists to provide comprehensive care tailored to each patient's specific needs. Each member of the care team contributes his or her expertise to ensure that care is coordinated, comprehensive and meets the requirements of a complex medical situation.

Chapter 4

Managing complications in hematology

Infections: increased vigilance in immunocompromised patients
Identifying signs of infection, managing additional precautions.

Identifying signs of infection in haematology patients is a top priority, as these patients, often immunocompromised due to disease or treatments such as chemotherapy or bone marrow transplants, are particularly vulnerable to infection. An infection, even a benign one in a healthy person, can rapidly become serious or even fatal in these patients. The ability to detect signs of infection at an early stage, as well as managing additional precautions to prevent the spread of germs, are therefore essential responsibilities for the nursing auxiliary.

Identifying **signs of infection** starts with rigorous daily clinical monitoring. One of the first indicators of infection is often a **fever**, even a mild one. In patients with bone marrow failure or undergoing intensive treatment, a body temperature above 38°C is already a cause for concern and should be reported immediately, as it may indicate the onset of infection. It's important to note that in some severely immunocompromised patients, the infection may not be accompanied by an obvious fever, making monitoring for other signs even more crucial.

In addition to temperature, the caregiver should be alert to other signs of **generalized** infection, such as **chills, excessive sweating, accelerated heart rate** (tachycardia) or **unexplained fatigue**. These manifestations, though sometimes discreet, can be early clues to a developing systemic infection. Similarly, specific symptoms such as **persistent cough** or shortness of breath may suggest a respiratory infection, while abdominal pain, diarrhea or vomiting may indicate a gastrointestinal infection.

It's also essential to monitor **the insertion sites of medical devices,** such as catheters or implantable chambers, which are prime entry points for infections. Redness, swelling, localized warmth or purulent discharge around the insertion site are all warning signs that should be reported immediately, as they may reveal a local infection that could rapidly spread into the bloodstream.

When any of these signs are detected, the caregiver must quickly inform the medical team to enable rapid intervention. Infections can progress very rapidly in immunocompromised patients, and delayed management can lead to serious complications, such as sepsis. It is therefore imperative that any suspicion of infection is taken seriously and treated without delay.

In addition to identifying infections, the nursing auxiliary has a crucial role to play in **managing complementary precautions**, which are specific measures put in place to limit the spread of infections, both within the department and among other patients. These precautions vary according to the type of infection suspected or confirmed, but generally include several levels of protection.

Standard precautions consist of systematically applying reinforced hygiene measures for any contact with the patient or his or her environment. This includes hand washing with hydroalcoholic solutions before and after each interaction with the patient, and the use of gloves, masks and gowns when necessary. In some cases, more stringent precautions, known as **isolation precautions**, must be applied to prevent transmission of certain germs by air, droplets or direct contact. This may involve complete isolation of the patient in a dedicated room, equipped with air filtration systems, where access is limited and strictly supervised.

The caregiver ensures that all members of the care team, as well as visitors, comply with these strict isolation and disinfection protocols. This includes wearing specific outfits, limiting comings and goings in the patient's room, and regular cleaning and disinfection of surfaces touched by the patient. These measures are particularly important in preventing the spread of nosocomial infections (hospital-acquired infections), which represent a major hazard for haematology patients.

49

Another key aspect of supplementary precautions is the management of **medical waste and soiled linen**, which must be handled with care to avoid cross-contamination. Caregivers ensure that this waste is disposed of in accordance with current protocols, using single-use bags and ensuring that potentially contaminated equipment does not come into contact with other surfaces.

In some cases, patients with infections require special care and monitoring in terms of **nutrition** and **hydration**, as infection can further weaken an already fragile body. In such cases, the caregiver is responsible for ensuring that the patient eats properly and receives sufficient fluids to avoid dehydration, while adapting the diet to the patient's digestive tolerance.

Finally, an often overlooked but essential aspect of the management of supplementary precautions is the **education of the patient and those close to him or her**. Caregivers play an important role in explaining the measures to be followed to minimize the risk of infection, particularly for patients who have to return home after hospitalization. He or she informs patients and their families of the steps to take (such as regular hand-washing, wearing a mask, avoiding public places) and the precautions to take in their daily environment to avoid contamination. This not only reinforces the patient's safety in hospital, but also ensures that this vigilance continues when they return home.

Hemorrhage and other hematological emergencies
Recognition of signs of internal or external bleeding, rapid management.

Recognizing the signs of hemorrhage, whether internal or external, in hematology patients is a crucial task requiring constant vigilance. Patients with hematological diseases, particularly those undergoing chemotherapy or bone marrow transplants, are often at high risk of bleeding due to thrombocytopenia (low platelet count) or coagulation disorders. These patients may present with internal or external bleeding that is difficult to detect at first, but whose rapid management is essential to avoid serious or even fatal complications.

Recognizing the signs of external bleeding is more straightforward, but still requires careful observation. External bleeding manifests itself as visible bleeding, such as epistaxis (nosebleeds), gingivorrhagia (bleeding from the gums) or prolonged bleeding following a wound or injection. These symptoms must be taken very seriously, even if they seem minor, as a patient with thrombocytopenia may bleed profusely from small lesions or easily irritated areas. The caregiver must be particularly vigilant to these signs during daily hygiene or mouth care, monitoring the gums and taking precautions to avoid causing bleeding when brushing or handling teeth.

Other external signs, such as the appearance of bruises (spontaneous hematomas) on the skin without any apparent trauma, are also indicators of subcutaneous bleeding. These bruises, often diffuse and multiple, indicate that the body is bleeding under the skin, and their appearance should immediately alert the caregiver. The skin is a precious barrier, and these hematomas reflect a high degree of vascular fragility due to a drop in platelets, which calls for increased attention.

More subtle, **signs of internal bleeding** are often harder to spot, as they are not necessarily accompanied by immediate external manifestations. However, several clinical indicators can reveal that internal bleeding is occurring. Symptoms may include sudden pallor, cold sweats, a feeling of weakness or dizziness, and tachycardia (increased heart rate), as the body attempts to compensate for blood loss by increasing cardiac output. The patient may also experience abdominal or chest pain, intense headaches, or a sudden drop in blood pressure, all signs that blood is accumulating in an internal cavity.

More specific signs depend on the location of the internal bleeding. For example, a patient suffering from gastrointestinal haemorrhage may present with black, tarry stools (melena) or vomit blood (haematemesis). Cerebral haemorrhage, on the other hand, may manifest itself as impaired consciousness, sudden and severe headaches, or neurological disorders such as muscle weakness or blurred vision. In all these cases, prompt treatment is essential to prevent irreversible or fatal damage.

When a hemorrhage is suspected, **immediate management** is based on a number of coordinated actions. The caregiver plays a key role in detecting warning signs and alerting the medical team quickly. Effective communication is crucial to ensure a rapid, coordinated response to a potentially critical situation.

In the case of **external bleeding**, the first step is to try to control the bleeding. This may involve applying direct compression to the bleeding area, using a sterile compress or clean cloth. If the bleeding is severe, it's essential to maintain this pressure until the medical team can intervene. In the case of nasal bleeding, we recommend tilting the patient's head slightly forward and pinching the nose to try to stop the bleeding. If the bleeding is related to a medical device, such as a catheter, the site should be carefully inspected to ensure there is no significant leakage, and the healthcare team should be informed immediately.

In the case of **internal bleeding**, management requires rapid medical assessment, and often imaging or biological tests to localize the hemorrhage and assess its severity. However, before medical care arrives, the caregiver can help stabilize the patient by ensuring he or she remains supine, monitoring vital vitals (heart rate, blood pressure), and offering psychological support to reduce anxiety, which can worsen the situation.

One of the most common emergency treatments for hemorrhage in hematological patients is **platelet transfusion**. When bleeding is due to severe thrombocytopenia, platelet transfusion restores the blood's ability to clot and stops the bleeding. The caregiver plays an important role in preparing the patient for the transfusion, monitoring vital parameters before, during and after the procedure, and ensuring that everything runs smoothly and safely.

In addition to transfusion, haemostatic drugs may be administered to promote coagulation. The caregiver ensures that these treatments are administered as prescribed, and carefully monitors any potential side effects.

Finally, after the hemorrhage, the caregiver plays a role in monitoring and **preventing recurrence**. This includes extra vigilance regarding puncture sites, medical devices or any signs of infection that could further weaken blood vessels. It is also essential to limit unnecessary invasive procedures, such as intramuscular injections or repeated sampling, in patients at high risk of bleeding.

Treatment side effects: special monitoring
Chemotherapy, radiotherapy, immunotherapy: management of nausea, mucositis, extreme fatigue.

The management of patients undergoing chemotherapy, radiotherapy or immunotherapy requires special attention because of the severe side effects these treatments cause. Among these effects, nausea, mucositis and extreme fatigue are among the most frequent and distressing. They can have a considerable impact on patients' quality of life, both physically and emotionally, and require appropriate, ongoing and coordinated management. The nursing auxiliary plays an essential role in this management, being both a vigilant observer of the signs of these side effects, a support in the administration of care, and a sympathetic interlocutor for the patient.

Nausea and vomiting, often associated with chemotherapy, but also with radiotherapy and, in some cases, immunotherapy, are particularly disabling side effects. They are generally caused by irritation of the stomach cells and nerve centers responsible for the vomiting reflex. Management of nausea begins with prevention and administration of antiemetics, prescribed by the medical team to control these symptoms. However, these drugs are not always totally effective, and this is where the caregiver comes in to relieve the patient on a daily basis.

First of all, the caregiver must ensure that the patient takes his or her antiemetic medication before chemotherapy or radiotherapy, as prescribed. Next, it's important to adapt the patient's diet. Light, divided meals at room temperature can help reduce nausea. Foods that are fatty, spicy or too high in fiber should be avoided, as they can aggravate the feeling of nausea. In addition, patients should be encouraged to keep well hydrated by taking small sips of water or non-carbonated drinks throughout the day, as dehydration can exacerbate vomiting. The caregiver can also suggest non-medicinal methods, such as the use of ginger in herbal tea or candy form, which is recognized for its natural anti-emetic properties.

In addition to nausea, **mucositis**, or inflammation of the mucous membranes of the mouth and digestive tract, is another frequent side effect, particularly in patients undergoing chemotherapy and radiotherapy targeting the head, neck or digestive tract. Mucositis manifests as intense pain, ulceration and difficulty in eating, drinking and speaking, which can lead to undernutrition and great suffering for the patient.

Mucositis management is based on meticulous oral hygiene and the prevention of secondary infections. The caregiver ensures that the patient regularly performs antiseptic mouthwashes, using mild, non-irritating solutions to clean the mouth without aggravating lesions. Soft toothbrushes are preferred to avoid irritation of sensitive gums and mucous membranes, and the use of alcohol-containing products, which can dry out the mouth and accentuate pain, should be avoided.

Diet also plays an essential role in the management of mucositis. Patients should be encouraged to eat soft, easy-to-swallow foods, and to avoid spicy, acidic or excessively hot dishes, which can further irritate the mouth. In some cases, the administration of liquid nutritional supplements may be necessary to ensure adequate caloric intake when solid food becomes too painful.

Relieving the pain associated with mucositis is a priority, and the caregiver must be attentive to the patient's complaints about oral pain. If pain is severe, topical analgesics or local anesthetic solutions can be offered before meals, to enable the patient to eat with less discomfort. Collaboration with the nursing and medical team is essential to adjust pain management to the patient's needs.

Extreme fatigue, or asthenia, is another major side effect of oncology treatments. It is often described by patients as a deep, overwhelming fatigue that does not go away with rest. This fatigue can be caused by chemotherapy-induced anemia, damage to healthy tissue during radiation therapy, or excessive activation of the immune system during immunotherapy treatments.

To manage this fatigue, the caregiver plays a key role in encouraging the patient to balance activity and rest periods. It is often necessary to readjust the patient's daily routine to avoid exhaustion caused by trying to maintain his or her usual level of activity. An adapted rhythm, alternating light activities and rest periods, can help to better manage exhaustion. Patients should be encouraged to listen to their bodies, and not to force themselves when they feel too tired.

Nutrition and hydration are also important in managing fatigue. The caregiver can ensure that the patient receives balanced, nutrient-rich meals to support the body during treatment. In addition, good hydration is crucial, as dehydration can exacerbate fatigue.

Psychological support is an equally essential aspect of fatigue management. Extreme fatigue can have significant emotional repercussions, plunging some patients into feelings of helplessness or depression. By listening attentively and providing support, the caregiver can help the patient to express these feelings, normalize these emotions, and reassure him or her that fatigue is part of the healing process. This moral support is often just as important as the physical interventions, helping to preserve the patient's psychological well-being, even in the most difficult of times.

Finally, it is essential that the caregiver works **closely with the multidisciplinary team**, including doctors, nurses, dieticians and psychologists, to ensure comprehensive care tailored to each patient's specific needs. Each treatment, each patient, and each side effect requires an individualized, coordinated approach to provide the best possible care.

Chapter 5

Helping and communicating with hematology patients

Active listening and non-verbal communication with frail patients
Listening and communication techniques to reassure and establish a relationship of trust.

Listening and communication skills are at the heart of the nursing assistant's profession, particularly in haematology, where patients, often faced with serious illnesses and long, demanding treatments, experience considerable anxiety. In this context, the ability to reassure patients and establish a relationship of trust is crucial to their physical and psychological well-being. Effective, empathetic communication is not just about exchanging information; it also involves active listening, respectful dialogue and constant support, so that the patient feels understood, supported and secure.

Active listening is an essential first technique in establishing a relationship of trust. It goes beyond simply hearing what the patient is saying. It involves focusing fully on the patient's words, showing that their concerns are being taken seriously, and responding appropriately to their needs, whether verbal or non-verbal. This may involve maintaining benevolent eye contact, nodding to show that you're following the thread of the conversation, and using expressions that encourage the patient to continue speaking, such as simple phrases like "I understand", or "Can you tell me more?".

In active listening, it's also important to pay attention to the patient's **body language**. Indeed, many patients, especially those who are tired, stressed or in pain, may not verbalize their concerns or pain directly. A patient who tenses up, looks away or withdraws may be expressing fears or discomfort without articulating them. By observing these non-verbal cues, the caregiver can provide an opening to discuss these concerns, by asking gentle, non-intrusive questions such as: "You seem worried, do you want to talk about it?" or "How are you feeling at the moment?".

Reformulation is another powerful technique for establishing a relationship of trust. Rephrasing consists in taking the patient's words and echoing them back to caregiver the, to make sure you've understood what he or she is saying. For example, if a patient says: "I'm really exhausted, I don't know if I'm going to make it", the caregiver might reply: "You're feeling very tired and that worries you, isn't it? This technique allows the patient to feel heard and understood, while encouraging him or her to go deeper into their feelings or clarify their needs. It also demonstrates to the other person that the caregiver is fully engaged in the exchange, and takes the patient's concerns to heart.

In addition to active listening and rephrasing, **non-verbal communication** is a powerful tool for reassuring a patient. Simple gestures such as placing a hand on the shoulder, gently adjusting a pillow or offering a kind smile can bring great comfort. These small gestures show patients that they are being cared for not only medically, but also in human terms. They create a climate of trust and serenity, reducing the anxiety that often accompanies heavy treatment or moments of uncertainty.

Clear communication is also essential to reassure patients. In hematology, treatment and care can be complex, and it's not uncommon for patients to feel overwhelmed by the flood of information. The caregiver can play a mediating role, explaining in a simple and accessible way what is going to happen, what the forthcoming treatment or care consists of, and why it is necessary. Using clear language, avoiding overly technical medical terms, and giving the patient the opportunity to ask questions all help to reduce anxiety and reinforce their sense of control over their own situation.

One of the keys to good communication is to **leave room for silence**. Sometimes, patients simply need time to assimilate information, express their emotions or reflect. The caregiver needs to be comfortable with these moments of silence, which can be very emotionally productive. These moments allow the patient to refocus, to gather their thoughts, and to feel that we are at their side, ready to listen without haste. Silence can also serve as a doorway for the patient to share concerns or feelings they might not otherwise have expressed.

Another dimension of trust-building communication is **consideration of the patient's autonomy**. The patient needs to feel that he or she is an actor in his or her own care, and not simply an object of treatment. This means asking open-ended questions such as "How would you like us to proceed?" or "Are there things you'd like us to do differently?". Involving patients in their care, even in seemingly innocuous details, gives them a sense of control over their situation, which is reassuring in a medical environment often perceived as controlled and rigid. It also shows patients that their individual needs and preferences are respected and taken into account.

Finally, it's important to cultivate **patience and empathy**. Every patient reacts differently to illness, treatment and the hospital environment. Some are very anxious, while others may be irritable or closed to communication. In these situations, the caregiver must remain patient, empathetic and understanding. Empathy is the ability to put oneself in the patient's shoes, to understand their experience without judging them, and to adapt one's attitude to the specific needs of each individual. This quality is essential for creating a lasting relationship of trust, as it shows patients that they are understood not only in their physical pain, but also in their emotions and doubts.

Managing the announcement and providing support at the end of life.
The caregiver's role with palliative care patients and support for families.

The caregiver's role with palliative care patients is one of depth and humanity, accompanying people at the end of life with dignity, respect and kindness. In palliative care, the aim is no longer to cure, but to provide maximum comfort, pain relief and physical, emotional and spiritual support for both patient and family. This holistic approach to care requires not only technical skills, but above all a great deal of human sensitivity, listening skills and a comforting presence.

When a patient enters the palliative phase, the caregiver becomes a **key player in physical comfort**. Care is geared towards improving quality of life, even if the disease can no longer be treated curatively. The caregiver provides daily hygiene care, such as washing and body care, ensuring that these gestures are performed with gentleness and respect, as the patient's body can be particularly fragile and sensitive. Each gesture is carried out with particular care to avoid any additional pain or discomfort. For example, mobilization must be gentle and appropriate, and regular position changes are designed to prevent bedsores and other complications associated with immobility.

One of the most important aspects of palliative care is **pain management**. The caregiver plays a fundamental role in the daily assessment of the patient's pain. He/she observes facial expressions, postures and non-verbal reactions that may indicate suffering, even when the patient can no longer express /him herself clearly. In collaboration with the nursing and medical team, he/she participates in the administration of analgesic treatments, whether medicinal or non-medicinal, and monitors their effectiveness. Palliative care also includes comfort techniques, such as light massage, the application of hot or cold compresses, or the use of cushions to relieve pressure points. The caregiver, through his or her daily proximity to the patient, becomes one of the first points of reference to signal any changes in the patient's pain or comfort, enabling rapid adaptation of treatment.

Beyond physical care, **emotional support** is at the heart of the palliative care caregiver's mission. Patients at the end of life experience moments of great vulnerability, marked by fear of death, uncertainty about the future and sometimes profound loneliness. The caregiver's regular, reassuring presence becomes an indispensable source of moral support. He or she is often the one who spends the most time with the patient, listening to his or her fears, memories or unexpressed needs. Listening, in this context, is essential. It's not a question of trying to provide answers or solutions, but of offering an attentive ear, accepting silences, and accompanying the patient with kindness in his final moments.

In this approach, **respect for patient autonomy** is paramount. Even at the end of life, each patient must retain some control over his or her care and decisions. The caregiver ensures that the patient's wishes are respected, whether they concern small daily preferences (such as the position in which he or she prefers to rest, or the foods he or she can still tolerate) or more important end-of-life decisions. By maintaining this autonomy, the caregiver helps to offer the patient precious dignity at a time when so much control over life is slipping away.

Palliative care not only concerns the patient, but also his or her **loved ones and family**, who are also going through a difficult period. Families often find themselves at a loss when faced with the illness and imminent death of their loved one, and the caregiver becomes a privileged interlocutor to reassure, inform and support them. The caregiver can act as a **mediator**, explaining care procedures to the family, clarifying certain medical aspects that are sometimes difficult to understand, or simply offering a comforting presence. He or she is there to answer their questions, allay their fears and help them understand the end-of-life process, while involving them in the care if they so wish.

Managing family emotions is another important component. Family members may go through phases of anger, sadness, incomprehension or denial. By listening empathetically, the caregiver enables them to express their feelings without judgment. Sometimes, words are insufficient or useless, and the caregiver's simple reassuring presence is enough to bring comfort in moments of great emotional pain. He or she is also attentive to family dynamics, respecting the different rhythms and ways of coping that each person may have.

In palliative care, the caregiver also assists the family in the **anticipated mourning process**. The end of life is an intense time, marked by the need for emotional preparation for the loss of a loved one. The caregiver helps loved ones to create meaningful moments of exchange with the patient, to find space for a serene farewell, and to express emotions that are sometimes buried. They can facilitate visits, offer moments of intimacy and respect each family's needs in terms of rituals or spiritual support.

Finally, **post-mortem support** is also a delicate but essential mission for the caregiver. After the patient's death, the caregiver helps the family through the initial stages of bereavement. They care for the body with great dignity, respecting the family's religious or cultural beliefs and rituals, and provide a peaceful setting for the final farewell. These moments, marked by respect and discretion, are crucial to enabling loved ones to grieve in respectful and humane conditions.

Ethics and respect for patient dignity
Ethical issues related to hematology care, including respect for consent and confidentiality.

The ethical issues involved in haematology care are particularly sensitive because of the complexity of treatments, the seriousness of the diseases, and the vulnerability of patients who are often faced with difficult choices. Among these issues, respect for **informed consent** and **confidentiality** occupy a central place. These principles are not only legal obligations, but also the foundations of the relationship of trust between the patient, the healthcare team and the medical institution. They help to ensure that care is not only effective, but also respectful of patients' rights, dignity and autonomy.

Informed consent is a cornerstone of medical ethics, and is particularly important in hematology, where treatments can be heavy, complex and with potentially serious consequences. Patients with hematological diseases, such as leukemia, lymphoma or myeloma, are often faced with critical decisions about their treatment, which may include intensive chemotherapy, bone marrow or stem cell transplants, and other high-risk interventions. These treatments carry significant side effects, risks of complications, and sometimes uncertain outcomes. It is therefore essential that patients are fully informed of these risks and expected benefits before giving their consent.

For consent to be truly informed, the patient must receive clear, precise and comprehensible information about his or her state of health, the treatment options available, and the implications of each choice. The caregiver, although not in charge of the initial medical discussion, plays a crucial role in this process by helping to clarify certain practical or technical aspects of care. They can also answer patients' questions about the day-to-day consequences of treatment, such as how it will affect their comfort, mobility or ability to carry out their usual activities. The caregiver is often the one who explains in simple terms the procedures the patient will undergo, enabling him or her to better understand and feel more comfortable with the decisions to be made.

Respect for **consent** also implies that the patient has the possibility of **refusing** treatment or changing his or her mind at any time. This can be particularly difficult in haematology, where stopping treatment can have serious consequences. However, it is essential that the patient retains this freedom of choice, even at times when medical pressure is high. The caregiver, by listening attentively and being present regularly, can play an important role in relaying the patient's doubts or anxieties to the nursing team. They are on the front line in detecting signs of distress or hesitation, and can help facilitate a more in-depth discussion between patient and doctor to re-evaluate treatment options.

Confidentiality is another major ethical issue in hematology care. Information relating to a patient's state of health, treatment and medical data must be protected with the utmost care. In haematology, where patients may be hospitalized for long periods and undergo multiple consultations and exchanges between healthcare professionals, data confidentiality can sometimes be put to the test. Like all members of the healthcare team, orderlies are bound by professional secrecy. This means that under no circumstances may they divulge patient information to unauthorized third parties, be they relatives or other caregivers not directly involved in the patient's care.

The management of patient information requires particular vigilance. When information is transmitted between teams, whether orally or in writing, it is imperative to ensure that only those directly involved in the patient's care have access to this data. The nursing auxiliary plays an active part in this protection by ensuring that discussions about the patient take place in a confidential setting, and by guaranteeing that medical documents are not left unattended.

Respect for confidentiality also goes beyond the simple protection of medical data. It includes respect for the patient's privacy in the context of the treatment itself. This means that care procedures must be carried out with discretion, respecting the patient's modesty. When hygiene care or physical examinations are carried out, the caregiver must always take care to preserve the patient's privacy, by closing the door, using screens, and covering the patient as much as possible to avoid unnecessary exposure. These small attentions are essential to ensure that the patient feels respected and protected, even at moments of great vulnerability.

The ethical aspect of **respecting** patient **beliefs and preferences** is also central to hematology care. Every patient has values, religious beliefs or personal preferences that must be taken into account when planning care. For example, some patients may refuse certain medical interventions for religious or ethical reasons, such as blood transfusions or certain types of treatment.

By listening to these preferences, the caregiver helps to adapt care to respect the patient's wishes, while maintaining the quality and safety of care.

It's also important to stress that respect for confidentiality and consent extends to support for families. In hematology, the patient's loved ones often play a central role in providing emotional and practical support. However, the caregiver must navigate carefully to ensure that information shared with families respects the patient's wishes. Patients may not wish to disclose certain information about their condition or treatment to their loved ones, and this wish must be respected. In such cases, the caregiver must use tact and discretion to ensure that discussions with the family do not compromise the patient's confidentiality.

Finally, **ethical decisions** about end-of-life care, particularly palliative care, can raise complex issues of consent and confidentiality. Terminally ill patients may express wishes concerning the cessation of treatment or the way in which they wish to be accompanied in their final moments. It is essential that these wishes are respected, and the caregiver plays a supportive role in these situations, ensuring that the patient's decisions are clearly communicated and respected by the entire care team.

Chapter 6

Interprofessional collaboration in hematology

The caregiver's central role in the care team
The caregiver as intermediary between patient, nurse and doctor.

As the intermediary between patient, nurse and doctor, the nursing auxiliary plays a key role in the care chain. This role goes beyond the simple execution of technical or assistance tasks: it involves ensuring fluid communication between all those involved in the care process, while ensuring the patient's well-being. The caregiver thus becomes a **bridge between the different dimensions of care**, providing the continuity and coherence that are essential to quality care.

As the caregiver is closest to the patient in daily acts of care, he or she is often the one who spends the most time with the patient. As such, they are the first to **observe subtle changes** in the patient's physical or emotional state. Whether it's a change in temperature, unusual fatigue, increased pain, or a simple change in behavior, the caregiver is able to pick up on these signals quickly. This observation role is fundamental, as it enables **this information to** be **passed on** to nurses and doctors accurately and in real time. For example, if they notice swelling around a catheter or redness on the skin, they immediately inform the nurse, who can assess the situation and, if necessary, intervene or alert the doctor to adjust treatments or carry out further tests.

As an intermediary, the nursing auxiliary also ensures the **smooth transmission of information** during team handovers. Hospital care, particularly in hematology, is often complex and involves multidisciplinary teams. During team changes, orderlies play a crucial role in ensuring that the relevant information on the patient's condition, feelings and care is passed on to their colleagues. This continuity is essential to avoid errors or omissions that could affect the quality of care or patient safety. The nursing auxiliary must therefore be able to synthesize information clearly and precisely, highlighting critical points, while ensuring that every necessary detail is conveyed correctly.

In addition to their role of observation and transmission, orderlies are often the ones who **facilitate communication between the patient and other members of the medical team**. Patients, especially those hospitalized for long periods or suffering from serious illnesses, often feel intimidated by doctors, or hesitate to express certain concerns, whether for fear of disturbing them or because they find it difficult to articulate their worries. The caregiver, through daily contact and attentive listening, becomes a **privileged interlocutor**, able to understand the patient's anxieties, pain or unexpressed needs. He or she can then relay this information to nurses or doctors, so that care can be tailored to the patient's real needs.

This intermediary role is particularly important when medical decisions have to be made. By acting as a link between the patient and the health-care team, the caregiver helps to **clarify exchanges** and ensure that the patient has fully understood the information conveyed by doctors or nurses. If the patient is confused about a treatment or procedure, the caregiver can re-explain in simple terms what is expected, or escalate the patient's questions to the doctor, ensuring that the latter takes the time to address the patient's concerns. This role is crucial in ensuring that informed consent is respected, as it ensures that the patient has all the information he or she needs to make informed decisions.

The nursing auxiliary also acts as a **valuable relay for the nursing team**, performing certain acts under their supervision, enabling nurses to concentrate on more technical or administrative tasks. For example, the caregiver may be responsible for monitoring vital signs, preparing the patient for an examination, performing hygiene care, changing simple dressings or monitoring the side effects of certain treatments. By regularly transmitting information relating to such care, the nursing auxiliary contributes to the overall care of the patient, while lightening the nurse's workload.

This **relay role** is particularly visible during technical care or medical interventions. For example, before a medical procedure or examination, the orderly prepares the patient, informs him or her of the procedure and makes sure that he or she is comfortable. After the procedure, they monitor the patient's condition, looking for signs of potential complications, and pass on this information to the nurse or doctor. This vigilance and ability to anticipate the patient's needs enables better coordination of care and enhances patient safety and comfort.

As an intermediary, the nursing auxiliary also plays an important role in the **emotional care of** the patient. While doctors and nurses often focus on the clinical aspects of care, the caregiver, through his or her constant presence, is often the one who provides moral support to the patient, accompanying him or her in moments of doubt, anxiety or suffering. By taking the time to listen to patients, reassure them and answer their questions, the caregiver creates a bond of trust that enables patients to feel safe and supported, despite the seriousness of their illness. They also pass on this information to the nurses and doctors, so that the care team can adjust its approach to the patient's emotional needs.

Working in synergy with nurses, doctors and other professionals

The importance of effective communication in managing care and coordinating actions.

Effective communication is central to managing care and coordinating actions within a medical team. It is the key to ensuring the safety, quality and continuity of care, particularly in environments as complex as hematology departments. Well-mastered communication enables every member of the healthcare team to be informed of the patient's needs and condition, and to make informed decisions quickly and consistently. Without clear and precise communication, the risk of errors, misunderstandings or malfunctions increases considerably, to the detriment of the patient's well-being and safety.

The first step to effective communication in the medical environment is the **transmission of accurate and relevant information** concerning the patient's state of health. Every member of the team, whether caregivers, nurses, doctors or other healthcare professionals, must be able to share and receive accurate, up-to-date information on the care provided, ongoing treatments, any complications or changes in the patient's clinical condition. This includes objective data such as vital signs, but also more subjective observations on the patient's general well-being, comfort or anxieties.

The caregiver, for example, is often at the forefront of observing subtle signs of a change in the patient's condition, such as increased pain, increased fatigue, or a change in mood. It is essential that these observations are quickly shared with nurses and doctors, so that care can be adjusted accordingly. The caregiver's ability to **communicate** this information **effectively**, using clear language and emphasizing critical aspects, helps prevent potential signs of deterioration from going unnoticed. In return, the caregiver must also receive clear and precise instructions from nurses and doctors, to ensure that the care provided complies with medical protocols and team expectations.

Transmissions between teams, particularly when there is a change of shift, are particularly sensitive moments for communication. These transition periods must be carefully organized, as they determine the continuity of care and enable the new team to be immediately informed of recent developments concerning the patient. Effective communication is more than just a summary of actions taken; it must include a full update on clinical status, current treatments, problems encountered and planned interventions. During these transmissions, every detail counts: an oversight or misunderstood information can lead to errors or delays in care.

In addition to verbal transmissions, **written documentation** plays a crucial role in the communication of care. The patient's medical record is a central tool for recording all essential information on his or her state of health, treatments, test results and clinical decisions. Every intervention, observation or change in treatment must be clearly and accurately recorded by the entire health-care team. This sharing of information in written form enables all healthcare professionals to have access to a coherent and complete overview of the patient's situation, even in the absence of direct communication. A poorly filled-in, incomplete or imprecise file can lead to treatment errors or a poor assessment of the clinical situation.

Effective communication is not limited to the medical team; it also includes **dialogue with the patient** and, if necessary, his or her family. Patients need to be clearly informed about their illness, the treatments they are receiving, the tests they are scheduled to undergo, and the reasons for certain medical decisions. This transparency is essential to promote **informed consent** and to enable patients to understand and accept the care they are receiving. Complex medical terms must be translated into understandable language, and the patient must always have the opportunity to ask questions to dispel any doubts.

Similarly, smooth communication with the patient's family is crucial, especially when the patient is too debilitated to express his or her needs or fully understand the situation. Relatives need to be informed tactfully and sensitively of progress or complications, changes in treatment or critical decisions. They must also feel included in the care process, while respecting confidentiality and the patient's wishes. Good communication with the family helps to maintain a climate of trust, reduce anxiety and ensure that the care provided is in line with the wishes of the patient and his or her loved ones.

Coordinating actions within a multidisciplinary team also relies on effective communication. In haematology, where several specialties may be involved (haematologists, oncologists, nurses, care assistants, psychologists, nutritionists), cooperation between the various players is essential to ensure consistent, appropriate care. Everyone must have a clear understanding of their role and responsibilities, and be able to collaborate with other team members. This requires regular communication, both formal and informal, to ensure that everyone is working in the same direction, with the same care objectives.

The use of **multidisciplinary meetings** is an example of this necessary coordination. These meetings enable complex cases to be discussed, clinical situations to be analyzed, observations to be shared and joint treatment decisions to be made. Each team member can contribute his or her expertise and observations, and it is through open and respectful communication that the best decisions can be made. As a professional in direct contact with the patient, the caregiver can provide invaluable information on the patient's day-to-day condition, feelings or reactions to treatment, complementing the more technical data provided by doctors and nurses.

Staff meetings and passing on information
Key points to convey during team changes or multidisciplinary meetings.

Team changes and multidisciplinary meetings are crucial moments in care management, particularly in haematology where the complexity of treatments and the seriousness of pathologies require perfect coordination between the various healthcare professionals. At each changeover, the quality of care depends on clear, complete and relevant information being passed on, enabling the new team to take immediate charge of the patient without the risk of errors or loss of information. It is therefore essential to know what priority points need to be addressed during these transmissions, whether they take place as part of team changes or during multidisciplinary meetings.

The first fundamental point to convey concerns **the patient's current clinical condition**. This information includes a summary of changes in the patient's state of health since the last treatment, highlighting vital parameters (temperature, blood pressure, heart rate, oxygen saturation) and specific symptoms to watch out for, such as pain, fatigue, or any signs of infection or bleeding. For example, if a patient has developed a fever or sudden onset of pain, it is essential that the next team is informed so that monitoring can continue and care can be adjusted accordingly. Any recent change in the patient's state of health, however minor, should be mentioned, as it could signal a deterioration requiring rapid intervention.

Next, it's imperative to **take stock of current treatments**. This includes both drug treatments (chemotherapy, antibiotics, analgesics, infusions) and specific care (dressings, oxygen therapy, etc.). The orderly or nurse making the transmission must clearly indicate the treatments administered, those pending, and any recent adjustments, such as a change in dosage or the introduction of a new drug. It is also important to mention the **patient's reactions to treatment**, whether these be improvement, notable side effects or poor tolerance. In the case of a complex protocol, the timescales or methods of administration must be explicitly detailed to avoid any errors.

Upcoming examinations and procedures are also a central point of communication. Whether it's a blood test, imaging, biopsy or planned surgery, the next team needs to know what's planned for the patient. It is essential to specify the time, any specific instructions (fasting, hydration, etc.), and any other logistical elements. If the examination or procedure has already taken place, it is important to transmit the results obtained, or failing that, to indicate that the results are pending and how they might impact on the management.

Another key point is what **signs to look out for**. In the case of patients with haematological diseases, complications can arise unpredictably. It is therefore essential to inform the team taking over of the specific signs to watch out for. For example, in the case of a patient suffering from bone marrow aplasia, vigilance

74

for signs of infection (fever, chills, altered general condition) must be reinforced. In a patient on anticoagulants, signs of hemorrhage (hematomas, bleeding from the gums or nose, black stools) must be particularly closely monitored. By mentioning these elements, the next team knows exactly what to look out for, so they can act quickly if necessary.

An often overlooked but crucial aspect to convey is the **patient's emotional and psychological state**. Patients suffering from serious illnesses, such as those in haematology, often experience significant psychological distress. It is essential that the next team is informed of the patient's emotional state, whether this involves depressive symptoms, anxiety, or special needs for psychological support. If the patient has expressed fears or doubts during the previous relay, this information should be passed on so that the next team can adjust its approach and offer the necessary support. Relational and emotional aspects, although not always directly related to the disease, play a fundamental role in the overall support of the patient.

Information about family and friends is also important to communicate. This may include whether a relative has come to visit and expressed particular concerns, or whether important discussions have taken place with the family regarding health status or treatment decisions. In some cases, families may be emotionally distressed and need special support too. Informing the next team of the relationship between the patient and his or her loved ones helps to maintain continuity of care and avoid any break in the support provided to the family.

At **multidisciplinary meetings**, where the various members of the healthcare team (doctors, nurses, care assistants, psychologists, dieticians) come together to discuss complex cases, it is essential to give a complete overview of the patient's care pathway. Each discipline brings a different perspective to the patient's condition. The caregiver's daily contact with the patient can provide valuable information on aspects not directly perceived by other professionals: how the patient reacts to care,

75

whether he or she expresses particular needs in terms of comfort or nutrition, whether he or she seems morally affected by treatment, or whether he or she shows signs of non-verbalized distress. This information, which is often subtle, enables the medical team to tailor care to the patient's specific needs.

Finally, a central point not to be overlooked is the **coordination of the next stages of care**. Whether it's a change of team or a multidisciplinary meeting, it's important to clearly define the actions to be taken in the following hours or days. These actions may involve adjusting treatments, implementing new interventions, or adapting care based on recent test results. It is crucial that the next team knows exactly what is expected, to ensure continuity of care without disruption or delay.

Chapter 7

The emotional and psychological challenges of working in hematology

The emotional impact of serious illness on the caregiver
How to deal with feelings of sadness, helplessness or frustration in the face of illness.

Dealing with feelings of sadness, helplessness or frustration in the face of illness is an emotional challenge faced by many patients, particularly in specialties like hematology, where treatments can be long, painful and often uncertain. These emotions are natural, even inevitable, when a person is confronted with their own vulnerability, the uncertainty of the future or chronic pain. To help manage these feelings, it is essential to recognize and understand these emotions, while offering coping strategies that enable patients to find meaning and balance despite illness.

One of the first steps in dealing with sadness, helplessness and frustration is to **recognize that these emotions are legitimate**. In the face of a serious illness, it's normal to feel a profound sense of loss, whether it's the loss of a certain degree of autonomy, the loss of a life as it once was, or even the loss of certain physical abilities. These emotions must not be suppressed or ignored, as this could exacerbate the psychological distress. The caregiver, through active listening, can play a crucial role in validating these emotions, recognizing that the patient's suffering is real, and inviting them to express themselves without judgment. Providing this space for expression is often the first step in alleviating the emotional burden the patient is carrying.

Another way of managing these emotions is to **refocus attention on what can still be controlled**. One of the most frustrating factors for patients is the feeling of losing control over their bodies and their lives. The disease seems to dictate treatments, medical appointments, physical limitations, and this can be overwhelming. However, there are always aspects that the patient can control, even in the most difficult situations. These can include the way they choose to react to the disease, the small acts of self-care they can perform, or decisions about their daily lives (such as what they eat, how they spend their time, or how they manage their social interactions). **Giving patients back a**

measure of autonomy, however limited, can help them regain a sense of control and independence, reducing their perceived powerlessness.

Open communication with caregivers is also an essential element in managing negative emotions. Patients should feel free to share their concerns, doubts or frustrations with the medical team. If the patient feels lost in the face of treatment or disease progression, this can fuel feelings of helplessness and frustration. So it's crucial that patients are encouraged to ask questions, understand what's going on inside their bodies and express their feelings. The caregiver and other team members must be available to provide clear and appropriate explanations, enabling the patient to feel involved in his or her treatment, rather than passive.

The importance of **finding** outside **emotional support** should not be underestimated either. Patients may sometimes find it difficult to share their sadness or frustration with their families, for fear of worrying them or overloading them emotionally. So it's important that they can turn to professionals, such as psychologists or counselors, who are trained to support them through these difficult times. Support groups, where patients can talk to others in similar situations, can also provide a valuable space to share their feelings, find advice, or simply feel understood. The caregiver, who knows the patient well, can suggest such recourse according to individual needs, and facilitate contact with these services.

Another powerful tool for dealing with feelings of helplessness and frustration is to **seek personal meaning** through the ordeal of illness. For some, this may mean spiritual or religious introspection, while for others it may mean finding positive aspects or goals, even in difficult times. This can take the form of small personal projects that the patient can accomplish despite the illness, or acts of generosity, such as sharing their experience with other patients or providing support to those around them. Finding meaning in this experience often helps to transcend pain and frustration, giving a new perspective to the disease and the personal journey.

Managing emotional fatigue is also important in dealing with these feelings. Chronic illness, with its repeated treatments and constant ups and downs, can lead to mental and emotional exhaustion. It's important that patients are encouraged to take time out for themselves, to rest not only physically, but also mentally. Relaxation, meditation or mindfulness techniques can help to calm the mind and ease difficult emotions. The caregiver can suggest or facilitate access to these techniques, which have been proven to reduce illness-related stress and anxiety.

Finally, it's essential to **maintain social and emotional ties**. Sadness and helplessness can often lead to emotional isolation, with patients withdrawing into themselves. It is therefore crucial to ensure that patients remain connected to their loved ones, whether through regular visits or virtual exchanges. Emotional support from family and friends, even if it doesn't solve medical problems, can bring immense comfort. The caregiver can play a role in this dynamic, by encouraging visits or facilitating contact, while respecting the patient's rhythm and wishes.

Tools for managing stress and mental load
Relaxation and meditation techniques, and the importance of a healthy lifestyle.

Relaxation techniques, **meditation** and the importance of **healthy living** play a central role in supporting patients, particularly in medical contexts such as hematology, where illness and treatment can cause intense stress, heightened anxiety and physical and mental exhaustion. Although these approaches do not have a direct effect on the disease, they do offer powerful tools for managing psychological suffering, promoting recovery and improving the patient's overall quality of life. By integrating these practices into patients' daily lives, we can help them regain a sense of balance and well-being, despite the difficulties they face.

Relaxation techniques are simple but effective methods for calming the mind and relaxing the body. They involve inducing a state of muscular relaxation and mental tranquillity, which helps to reduce accumulated tension and alleviate stress. Among the most common techniques is **Jacobson's Progressive Relaxation**, based on progressive contraction and relaxation of muscle groups from head to toe. This method helps patients to become aware of their physical tensions and release them more effectively. By guiding the patient through this exercise, the caregiver can help him or her achieve a state of deep calm, conducive to recovery, particularly after a demanding treatment session.

Another popular relaxation technique is **controlled breathing**. It's a simple yet powerful approach, which involves focusing on the breath to regulate emotional state and reduce anxiety. By breathing slowly and deeply, the body activates the parasympathetic nervous system, responsible for relaxation and stress reduction. Encouraging the patient to take deep breaths, slowly inflating the abdomen on inhalation and exhaling for a long time, can rapidly induce a sense of calm. This method is particularly useful for patients who feel overwhelmed by anxiety or pain. The caregiver can show the patient how to integrate this technique into his or her daily routine, before treatment or during moments of stress, so that he or she can practice it independently.

Meditation is another approach that can have considerable effects on a patient's mental and physical well-being. Mindfulness meditation, in particular, is increasingly used in medical settings to help patients manage pain, anxiety and depression. This practice involves paying conscious, non-judgmental attention to the present moment. By concentrating on bodily sensations, breathing or the immediate environment, patients learn to observe their thoughts and emotions without getting caught up in them. This enables them to distance themselves from the anxieties associated with their illness, and better accept what cannot be changed.

In the medical context, meditation can also help **reduce the perception of pain**. Studies show that meditation alters the way the brain processes pain, making it less intense or intrusive. The caregiver can encourage the patient to try short moments of meditation, focusing on breathing or pleasant sensations, such as a positive mental image or comforting memory. With practice, even a few minutes of daily meditation can bring about a real improvement in the patient's emotional state, promoting relaxation and reducing stress.

In addition to relaxation and meditation techniques, **lifestyle** plays a fundamental role in the patient's ability to manage illness and promote healing. Hygiene of life encompasses several key aspects, including diet, sleep, exercise and the management of daily habits.

A **balanced diet** is essential to support the body in its healing process, especially in heavy treatments such as chemotherapy, which can considerably weaken the body. The caregiver can advise the patient to focus on foods rich in nutrients, vitamins and minerals, which boost the immune system and help combat fatigue. For example, fresh fruit and vegetables, lean proteins and complex carbohydrates are recommended to maintain energy levels. On the other hand, foods that are processed, fatty or rich in refined sugars may be inadvisable, as they fail to provide the body with the nutrients it needs. Hydration is also crucial, especially for patients undergoing chemotherapy, who need to compensate for fluid loss and avoid dehydration.

Sleep is another essential pillar of a healthy lifestyle. The body regenerates mainly during sleep, and sufficient rest is essential to cope with heavy treatment and disease-induced fatigue. Disturbed sleep can increase irritability, physical and mental fatigue, and reduce the body's ability to fight infection. The caregiver can encourage the patient to establish a regular sleep routine, avoid stimulants such as caffeine at the end of the day, and adopt soothing practices before bedtime, such as reading or relaxation. By fostering a calm, sleep-friendly environment, it is possible to improve the quality of rest and help the patient feel stronger in the face of treatment.

Moderate physical exercise, adapted to the patient's state of health, can also have positive effects. Even light physical activity, such as walking or stretching, keeps the body supple, strengthens muscles and stimulates the cardiovascular system. Exercise also releases endorphins, hormones that improve mood and provide a sense of well-being. It is therefore important for the caregiver to encourage, whenever possible, a certain amount of adapted physical activity, which can help reduce the feeling of chronic fatigue while improving the patient's morale.

Finally, **emotional balance** and the management of daily routines contribute to maintaining a healthy lifestyle. It is essential for patients to have moments of relaxation, leisure or social interaction, even in the hospital setting. These activities bring comfort and enable patients to reconnect with aspects of their lives that are not solely focused on their illness. The caregiver can help to arrange these moments, for example by facilitating family visits, creative activities or time for conversation.

The importance of peer support and ongoing training
The role of mutual support within the team and the importance of training to better cope with emotional challenges.

Mutual support within the healthcare team and the importance of **ongoing training** are two fundamental aspects of coping with the emotional challenges inherent in working in hematology, where the intensity of care, the severity of illness and proximity to critically ill patients can give rise to situations of considerable emotional stress. In this context, the ability to support each other, share difficulties encountered, and train regularly to better understand and manage these emotions, is essential to maintaining a strong, resilient team capable of delivering quality care.

Mutual support between colleagues is a pillar of cohesion in medical teams. Working in haematology, where care is often long, demanding and emotionally taxing, can put a strain on caregivers, whether they're nursing assistants, nurses or doctors. Daily interactions with patients who are going through critical moments in their lives, who are suffering, or who are sometimes at the end of their lives, create significant emotional tensions. In these circumstances, it's crucial that every member of the team feels supported by his or her peers, can express his or her feelings and share his or her difficulties without fear of judgment. This support takes the form of small, everyday gestures, such as taking the time to listen to a colleague after a difficult day, exchanging advice or practical solutions, or simply offering a moment's respite to someone who needs it.

Active listening between colleagues is a valuable tool for maintaining a climate of trust and caring. When caregivers feel able to talk about their emotions, frustrations or moments of doubt, they are better able to cope and recharge their batteries. Listening should not be seen as a weakness, but rather as a strength that enables everyone to better manage their emotional burden. By sharing their experiences, team members can also find comfort in the fact that they are not alone in feeling difficult emotions, helping them to better understand and accept them.

Teamwork in haematology also implies constant, fluid cooperation between the various members of the medical staff. Each caregiver brings his or her own expertise and sensitivity to the task, enabling comprehensive, holistic patient care. The importance of mutual support also lies in the ability to delegate or ask for help in the event of work overload or emotional difficulties. Times of complex care or end-of-life support can put a particular strain on caregivers, and it's at these times that team solidarity comes into its own. Knowing that you can count on your colleagues reduces the pressure on you, enabling you to concentrate fully on your tasks, with greater peace of mind and greater availability for the patient.

Ongoing training is another essential aspect of helping caregivers better manage the emotional challenges associated with their work. Training, whether technical or focused on emotional management, enables caregivers to develop new skills, deepen their understanding of pathologies and treatments, and better apprehend the stressful situations they encounter on a daily basis. Better mastery of care and therapeutic tools helps reduce the uncertainty and anxiety associated with complex care.

Training in **stress and emotional management** is particularly important. Knowing how to step back, recognize one's own limits and adopt stress management techniques is essential to prevent burnout, which is a very real risk in medical environments. Caregivers must learn to identify the signs of emotional overload and implement strategies to preserve their well-being. Training in **resilience** or **mindfulness meditation**, for example, enables caregivers to better manage moments of emotional tension, accept difficult situations, and focus on the positive aspects of their work.

Regular supervision or **discussion groups led** by psychologists can also provide a safe space where caregivers can freely discuss their emotions and experiences. These sessions enable them to take a step back from the situations they have experienced, gain a better understanding of the emotional mechanisms at play, and find solutions to improve the management of these emotions in their day-to-day work. They also provide an opportunity to strengthen the bonds between team members, to share common feelings and to support each other in moments of fatigue or doubt.

Finally, training must also include **awareness of ethical limits and patient autonomy**. Caregivers can sometimes feel frustrated when faced with situations in which they feel powerless, for example when the patient refuses treatment, or when the prognosis is bleak despite all efforts. Learning to respect the patient's autonomy, to accept that certain aspects are beyond their control, and to understand the ethical dynamics of end-of-life care, enables caregivers to cope better with these moments of helplessness. Training on these issues helps to develop a better understanding of the ethical issues at stake, and to accept that each patient has his or her own trajectory, which helps to reduce feelings of frustration or guilt among caregivers.

Chapter 8

Technological developments and their impact on the work of hematology nurses

New technologies in hematology: from artificial intelligence to care management software

Introducing the technologies that support caregivers in organizing care, monitoring patients and managing data (electronic patient records, remote monitoring systems).

Medical technologies are playing an increasingly crucial role in assisting caregivers, in particular, by enabling them to improve the organization of care, enhance patient monitoring and manage medical data more efficiently. With advances in technology, tools such as **electronic patient records (EPR)** and **remote monitoring** systems not only optimize the quality of care, but also ease the caregivers' workload by giving them access to accurate, real-time information, while simplifying coordination between the various members of the care team.

Electronic patient records (EPRs(are one of the most significant innovations in healthcare organization. These digital systems are gradually replacing paper records, centralizing all patient medical information in an easily accessible, searchable format. For the caregiver, this means instant access to the patient's medical history, current treatments, allergies, test results, as well as observations noted by doctors or nurses. This centralization of data enables **better care coordination**, as each member of the care team can consult and update the file in real time, reducing the risk of errors or omissions.

ECDs also enable caregivers to **better organize their daily work**. Thanks to these systems, he or she can consult assigned tasks, such as hygiene care, taking vitals, or administering treatments under the supervision of nurses. Automatic reminders integrated into the ECD ensure that scheduled care tasks, such as taking medication or changing dressings, are not forgotten, guaranteeing **better time management** and smoother organization of interventions. In addition, care assistants can enter their observations directly into the ECD, enabling smooth and immediate transmission of information to other team members, facilitating continuity of care during team changes.

Remote monitoring systems represent another significant technological advance that enhances the safety and quality of care. These technologies, often referred to as **telemonitoring** or **remote monitoring**, enable real-time monitoring of patient vitals without the need for a continuous physical presence at the bedside. For example, sensors placed on the patient's body continuously measure blood pressure, heart rate, oxygen saturation and temperature. These data are then transmitted to central software, which automatically alerts the nursing team to any anomalies, such as a drop in saturation or an acceleration in heart rate.

For the caregiver, these systems are a great help, as they enable **several patients to be monitored simultaneously** without having to be constantly present in each room. This frees up time for other tasks, while ensuring constant vigilance. If an alarm is triggered, the caregiver can intervene quickly or report the problem to the nurse or doctor, boosting responsiveness to emergencies. These monitoring systems are particularly useful for high-risk patients, such as those in intensive care or post-operative care, where rapid deterioration in health status can occur without immediate warning signs. Thanks to remote monitoring, caregivers can anticipate and prevent complications before they become critical.

Remote monitoring technologies also include **geolocation** devices for patients with reduced mobility or cognitive impairments, such as Alzheimer's patients. These devices can track patients' movements within the hospital or care home, and receive alerts if they leave secure areas. This type of technology helps to protect vulnerable patients while giving them greater autonomy, as caregivers don't need to monitor them all the time, but can intervene quickly if necessary.

Another benefit of technology for the caregiver is the management of **medications and treatments**. **Automated medication dispensers** are increasingly present in healthcare facilities. These systems ensure that the right doses of medication are administered at the right time to the right person, minimizing the risk of human error. These devices are often linked to electronic patient records, enabling medication administration to be tracked, and alerts to be sounded if medication is forgotten or not taken. This saves time and increases safety for the caregiver, who can follow treatment instructions without having to handle complex prescriptions directly.

Finally, managing **patient data** using digital technologies also helps to optimize the logistical aspects of care. For example, **inventory** management systems **for medical equipment** or pharmaceutical products are often interconnected with patient records and care protocols. This makes it possible to signal when a patient needs a specific treatment or material, while alerting the team to any shortage of resources. This automated management avoids stock-outs, guaranteeing constant availability of the resources needed for care to run smoothly.

The use of advanced medical devices: infusion pumps, vitals monitors, etc.
The importance for caregivers of mastering these devices to optimize the quality of care.

Caregivers' mastery of **technological devices** has now become essential to optimizing the quality of care in healthcare environments. With the rise of digital tools such as **electronic patient records**, **remote monitoring systems** and **automated medication dispensers**, caregivers must not only develop technical skills, but also integrate these devices into their daily practice to ensure more efficient, secure and patient-centered care.

One of the main reasons why mastery of these technologies is crucial is their ability to **improve care safety**. Devices such as electronic patient records (EPR) enable medical information to be centralized and updated in real time, reducing the risk of errors linked to incomplete or misinterpreted transmissions. By mastering the ECD, the caregiver can quickly access essential information such as allergies, current treatments or previous observations. This enables them to adjust their interventions to the patient's specific needs. For example, before administering any care or treatment, he or she can check the patient's history to ensure that there are no contraindications, thereby considerably improving **patient safety**.

In addition, mastery of technological devices contributes to **better organization of care**. Management systems integrated into ECDs enable caregivers to structure their daily work more fluidly and efficiently. He or she can consult the tasks assigned to each patient, monitor the progress of care, and receive reminders for upcoming interventions, whether for hygiene care, monitoring vitals, or administering medication. By optimizing time and resource management in this way, the caregiver is better able to devote greater attention to each patient, without the risk of delay or oversight. This **optimization of time is** particularly valuable in wards with heavy workloads, where care must be precisely coordinated between different healthcare professionals.

Remote monitoring systems, such as vital signs monitors, offer another opportunity for significant improvements in care, provided the caregiver knows how to use them effectively. These systems enable parameters such as blood pressure, heart rate or oxygen saturation to be monitored in real time, and alerts to be received in the event of anomalies. By mastering these devices, the caregiver can anticipate potential complications and react quickly, preventing the patient's condition from deteriorating without anyone noticing. The ability to **monitor several patients simultaneously** thanks to technology enhances vigilance while providing greater responsiveness in the event of a problem. It also enables better prioritization of interventions, concentrating resources where they are most needed.

The use of **automated medication dispensers** is another area where the caregiver's mastery of technology contributes directly to the quality of care. These devices ensure the safe dispensing of treatments by reducing human error in dose preparation. For a caregiver, knowing how to handle these devices correctly means ensuring that each patient receives the right dose of medication at the right time, in accordance with the medical prescription. Mastery of the traceability systems built into these devices also makes it possible to accurately track the administration of medication, and alert the team to any omissions or inconsistencies. This helps to reinforce **medication safety**, a critical issue in care management, particularly for patients suffering from serious pathologies such as haematological diseases, where treatments are often complex and potentially toxic.

In addition to the organizational and safety benefits, the caregiver's mastery of technology also promotes **smoother communication** between the various members of the care team. By using digital tools to record observations or update records, the caregiver facilitates the transfer of information between nurses, doctors and other caregivers. This fluid communication is essential to ensure **continuity of care**, particularly when teams change. For example, observations entered in the ECD enable the next team to take over without a break in information, thus reducing the risk of errors linked to incomplete oral transmissions or oversights. The centralization of data also enables each caregiver to have a **global and coherent view of** the patient's condition, thus reinforcing the quality and precision of interventions.

It's also important to emphasize that mastery of technology enables the caregiver to better accompany the patient and strengthen the **relationship of trust**. When technologies are used properly, they free up time and reduce errors, enabling the caregiver to concentrate more on the human aspect of care, such as listening, empathy and psychological support. What's more, by mastering digital devices, caregivers can explain to patients how the technologies used in their care work, helping to reassure them. For example, when a patient sees that his or her vital signs are continuously monitored by sensors, the caregiver can explain the process and answer any questions, offering **emotional support** in addition to medical monitoring.

Finally, **ongoing training** is essential to enable caregivers to fully master these constantly evolving technological tools. Innovations in digital healthcare are evolving rapidly, and it's essential that caregivers receive regular training to keep abreast of new features, system updates and new care management practices. Such training not only enhances the caregiver's efficiency, but also helps maintain a high level of **safety and quality of care**, ensuring that technologies are used optimally and in line with safety protocols.

Ongoing training and the need to adapt to technological change
How to keep abreast of emerging technologies and the importance of training in this field.

In an ever-changing medical environment, it's crucial for caregivers to keep up to date with the **emerging technologies** that are transforming the healthcare field. These technological advances, whether digital care management tools, monitoring devices or telemedicine innovations, bring significant benefits in terms of safety, efficiency and quality of care. However, to take full advantage of these innovations, it is essential that caregivers receive regular training and develop an active technological culture.

Staying abreast of emerging technologies requires **regular**, proactive **monitoring**. The healthcare sector is undergoing rapid change, with the introduction of new technologies designed to improve patient care, automate certain tasks and reduce errors. Caregivers can keep abreast of these developments by accessing specialized sources of information such as **medical journals, specialized health technology newspapers**, or **conferences** and **seminars** dedicated to technological innovations in healthcare. Taking part in these events not only allows you to discover the latest advances, but also to meet other professionals, share experiences and discuss best practices.

Ongoing training is at the heart of our strategy to keep abreast of these innovations. In a context where digital tools are rapidly evolving, specific training is essential to understand how new technologies work and how to integrate them into daily practice. Such training can be offered by healthcare establishments themselves, in the form of **in-house training sessions**, where new devices are explained and demonstrated by specialist trainers. In this way, caregivers can familiarize themselves with the technologies before they are introduced into their departments, thus avoiding errors of use or wasted time during initial trials.

Online platforms are also playing an increasingly important role in the continuing education of caregivers. Thanks to e-learning tools, caregivers can access remote training modules, at their own pace, on subjects as varied as electronic patient record (EPR) management, the use of connected monitoring devices or advances in telemedicine. These platforms often offer certifications, validating the skills acquired and contributing to continuing professional development. By regularly engaging in such training, caregivers keep abreast of the latest advances and can quickly integrate innovations into their practice.

One of the major benefits of keeping up to date with emerging technologies is the ability to **respond to changing patient needs** and **improve the quality of care**. For example, the introduction of telemonitoring enables caregivers to monitor patient vitals remotely, reducing the need for constant room visits and allowing attention to be focused on those patients most in need of immediate care. Similarly, mastering ECDs facilitates care management by providing instant, secure access to medical information, eliminating the risk of errors associated with miscommunication or incomplete records. Without regular training in these tools, caregivers could find themselves overwhelmed by the rapid pace of technological change, which would have a detrimental effect on the quality of patient care.

In addition to the practical benefits, keeping up to date with emerging technologies helps caregivers **gain confidence** in their work. When properly mastered, technology becomes a powerful ally, enabling them to work more efficiently and with greater peace of mind. It also reduces the mental workload associated with care, by automating certain tasks or facilitating data management. For example, medication management or care traceability systems help to reduce human error, saving time and providing peace of mind for the caregiver, who can concentrate on the relational and human aspects of his or her work.

It's also important to understand that continuing education on technologies should not be limited to the technical aspect, but should include reflections on **ethical implications** and **data security**. The use of technologies such as ECDs and monitoring systems involves the management of sensitive medical information. Caregivers therefore need to be trained not only in the use of these technologies, but also in protecting **patient confidentiality** and complying with security protocols to avoid any risk of data leakage or misuse. In addition, training addresses the ethical issues involved in automating care, to ensure that technology remains a tool at the service of the patient and does not replace the human interaction essential to the patient's psychological well-being.

Collaboration with other healthcare professionals is also essential to keep abreast of innovations. By working closely with nurses, doctors, health technicians and biomedical engineers, caregivers can not only learn directly from the experiences of their colleagues, but also share their own observations and concerns about the use of technology on a daily basis. These exchanges help to create a **collective learning culture**, where new practices are discussed, refined and gradually integrated.

Finally, it is important that caregivers are encouraged to **adopt a proactive attitude** to emerging technologies. Waiting for formal training should not dampen personal interest and curiosity about new technologies. Caregivers can take the initiative in testing digital tools, asking questions of their more experienced colleagues, or even requesting further training if they feel a technology could improve their efficiency or work comfort.

Chapter 9

Care of patients with rare diseases in hematology

Introduction to rare hematological diseases: sickle cell anemia, bone marrow failure, etc.
Presentation of the main rare diseases, their characteristics, and the particularities of their management.

Rare diseases are conditions that affect a small percentage of the population, generally defined as affecting less than one person in 2,000. Although individually rare, it is estimated that there are between 6,000 and 8,000 rare diseases, and together they affect millions of people worldwide. These diseases, often genetic in origin, are characterized by extreme clinical diversity, complex symptoms and often long and difficult treatment paths. The management of these diseases presents specific challenges due to the scarcity of available knowledge and treatments, requiring a highly specialized, multidisciplinary approach.

Among rare diseases, some are particularly well known and illustrate the challenges they represent. **Cystic fibrosis**, for example, is a rare genetic disease that mainly affects the respiratory and digestive tracts. It causes abnormal production of thick mucus, obstructing bronchial tubes and pancreatic ducts. Patients suffer from chronic cough, frequent lung infections and malabsorption of nutrients. Management of cystic fibrosis is based on multidisciplinary treatment, with antibiotics for infections, respiratory physiotherapy to facilitate mucus elimination, and pancreatic enzymes to improve digestion. Treatment is long and demanding, and requires regular monitoring to avoid serious complications such as respiratory failure.

Another rare disease is **Duchenne** muscular dystrophy, which mainly affects boys. This genetic disease causes progressive degeneration of skeletal, cardiac and respiratory muscles. The first symptoms generally appear in childhood, with muscular weakness leading progressively to loss of walking and damage to respiratory and cardiac muscles. Management of Duchenne muscular dystrophy includes drug treatments to slow disease progression (such as corticosteroids), physiotherapy to maintain

98

mobility, and surgery to treat orthopedic complications. Specialized respiratory care is also essential as the disease progresses.

Rare metabolic diseases, such as Fabry disease or phenylketonuria (PKU), represent another group of rare pathologies. **Fabry disease** is an inherited disorder caused by an accumulation of certain lipid substances in the cells, resulting in damage to the blood vessels, kidneys, heart and nervous system. Symptoms include neuropathic pain, kidney damage, heart disease and stroke. Treatment is based on enzyme replacement therapy, which aims to replace the missing enzyme to prevent accumulation of lipid substances and slow disease progression. Phenylketonuria, on the other hand, is a genetic disease that results in an inability to metabolize an amino acid called phenylalanine, leading to toxic accumulation in the body. Management is based on a strictly controlled diet, low in phenylalanine, to avoid severe neurological damage.

Rare cancers, although less frequent than more common forms such as breast or lung cancer, pose similar challenges in terms of diagnosis and treatment. **Ewing's sarcoma**, for example, is a rare bone tumor that mainly affects children and young adults. It manifests as bone pain and swelling around the tumor. Diagnosis of these rare cancers can be delayed, as initial symptoms are often vague or attributed to more benign causes, such as minor trauma. Management of Ewing's sarcoma relies on a combination of chemotherapy, radiotherapy and surgery, but often requires specific expertise in specialized pediatric oncology centers.

Spinal muscular atrophy is another rare disease that illustrates the challenges of care. It is a genetic neurodegenerative disease that affects the motor neurons responsible for muscle control. It results in progressive muscular atrophy, affecting breathing, swallowing and mobility. Management is complex and multidisciplinary, involving respiratory care, physiotherapy to maintain muscle function, and nutritional support treatments. Recently, innovative new treatments such as gene therapies have

99

brought considerable hope to spinal muscular atrophy patients, by altering the course of the disease.

Rare hematological diseases, such as **congenital amegakaryocytic thrombocytopenia** or **Fanconi anemia**, are also examples of rare pathologies requiring specialized care. Fanconi anemia is a genetic disease characterized by progressive failure of the bone marrow, responsible for blood cell production. Patients are at risk of developing leukemia or other cancers at an early age. Management often includes bone marrow transplants, and rigorous monitoring to prevent infections and treat hematological complications. Because of the genetic nature of these diseases, genetic counseling and family screening play a key role in their management.

The **particularity of care for rare diseases** lies in their complexity and the fact that they often require **multidisciplinary management**, involving specialists from different fields. The rarity of these diseases also means that many caregivers may be unfamiliar with the symptoms or specific treatment protocols. This calls for ongoing training and close coordination between care teams, often within centers of reference dedicated to rare diseases. These centers bring together multidisciplinary teams capable of offering specialized care and access to innovative or experimental treatments as part of **clinical research protocols**.

Another challenge is **access to treatments**. Drugs used to treat rare diseases are often **orphan drugs**, developed specifically for a restricted population, which can make access difficult due to their high cost or limited availability. Patients with rare diseases may also find it difficult to obtain a rapid diagnosis, due to the rarity of symptoms or lack of knowledge about the disease. This often leads to misdiagnosis, with an average delay of several years before the disease is identified.

Specific care for patients suffering from these pathologies
Specific needs in terms of hygiene, nutrition and psychological support for these patients.

Patients suffering from **rare diseases** have specific needs in terms of hygiene, nutrition and psychological support, due to the complexity and severity of their pathologies. These needs vary according to the particular symptoms of each disease, the evolution of the condition and the treatments received, but they always require individualized, multidisciplinary care. The aim is not only to guarantee optimal physical comfort, but also to take into account the emotional and psychological aspects, which are often profoundly affected by the disease.

Hygiene care

Hygiene care for patients with rare diseases can be particularly complex, due to the physical damage or invasive treatments they undergo. For example, certain diseases, such as muscular dystrophies (like Duchenne muscular dystrophy) or neurodegenerative diseases (like spinal muscular atrophy), lead to a progressive loss of mobility. These patients often require total assistance for hygiene care, including grooming, wound management, and prevention of skin complications such as pressure sores.

For these patients, daily hygiene is of paramount importance not only for their comfort, but also to prevent infections, which can have serious consequences due to the fragility of their condition. Caregivers must pay particular attention to the condition of the skin, ensuring that it is well moisturized and avoiding prolonged pressure on certain parts of the body. The use of specific equipment, such as anti-bedsore cushions, is often necessary to prevent complications linked to immobility.

In rare respiratory diseases, such as **cystic fibrosis**, hygiene care also includes specific gestures linked to airway maintenance. This includes regular respiratory physiotherapy sessions to clear mucus-clogged bronchial tubes. Preventing respiratory infections also involves strict hygiene, including frequent hand-washing, wearing masks in certain contexts, and disinfecting medical devices such as inhalers or ventilation machines.

Nutritional requirements

The **nutritional needs** of patients with rare diseases vary from pathology to pathology, but it is often necessary to follow specific diets to compensate for metabolic imbalances or digestive disorders associated with the disease. In some rare metabolic diseases, such as **phenylketonuria** or **Fabry disease**, dietary management is a key component of treatment. Phenylketonuria patients, for example, must follow a diet extremely low in phenylalanine, an amino acid their bodies cannot metabolize. Without such strict management, irreversible neurological damage can occur. Dietary support is therefore vital, and caregivers must be trained to understand these complex diets and ensure that patients and their families follow nutritional recommendations.

In rare diseases that affect digestive function, such as **cystic fibrosis**, nutritional supplements may be required to compensate for nutrient malabsorption. Cystic fibrosis patients often require enzyme supplements to aid fat and protein digestion, as well as increased caloric intake to compensate for energy losses linked to chronic inflammation and infection. High-calorie, nutrient-rich diets are often prescribed to help patients maintain adequate body weight, essential for their ability to fight infection and tolerate treatment.

On the other hand, patients suffering from **muscular dystrophy** or other neuromuscular diseases, who progressively lose the ability to feed themselves, may require more invasive **nutritional assistance**, such as feeding via gastric tube (gastrostomy) or intravenous infusion in the most severe cases. This management requires careful daily monitoring, as complications can arise, such as infections around gastrostomy devices, or difficulties in maintaining adequate electrolyte balance.

Psychological support

Psychological support for patients with rare diseases is an essential component of their overall care. These patients and their families often go through a profoundly destabilizing experience, marked by the uncertainty of diagnosis, the complexity of treatment, and sometimes medical wandering before adequate care is found. Dealing with the emotions associated with the rarity and severity of these diseases can lead to feelings of isolation, fear and powerlessness, both for patients and their families.

Children suffering from rare diseases, such as Duchenne muscular dystrophy or spinal muscular atrophy, face specific psychological challenges, particularly in terms of accepting increasing physical limitations and social integration. Psychological support must be designed to help the child understand his or her illness, accept the necessary adaptations to daily life, and maintain as normal a school and social life as possible. Psychological support can include individual sessions with a psychologist, as well as group approaches, enabling children to share their experiences with other young people in similar situations.

Adolescents and young adults with rare diseases can also face identity crises, as they have to reconcile their desire for autonomy with the reality of a disease that imposes significant limitations. Transitions to adulthood, particularly in terms of education, employment and interpersonal relationships, can be particularly complex. Psychological support adapted to this phase of life is crucial to help them project themselves into the future while managing medical challenges.

For **adults** with rare diseases, psychological support often takes on an existential dimension, linked to uncertain prognosis and increasing dependence on others. Patients can feel isolated, especially as little is known about their disease, even in the medical community. The need for regular psychological support, with professionals trained in the management of rare diseases, is essential to help these patients overcome the feelings of anxiety, frustration or depression that can result from the disease.

Finally, we must not overlook the psychological impact of rare diseases on **families**. Parents of children with rare diseases are often faced with an immense emotional burden, juggling complex care, treatment management, and the search for information that is sometimes difficult to obtain. Psychological support for the family, including support sessions and discussion groups, can help prevent exhaustion and improve the quality of family life. Offering parents a space for dialogue, where they can share their anxieties, frustrations and hopes, helps to alleviate the emotional burden that often accompanies these illnesses.

The challenges of research and innovative treatments for rare diseases
Therapeutic advances and challenges in the management of these diseases, particularly in the context of clinical trials.

Rare diseases pose particular challenges in terms of management, largely due to the lack of available treatments and the limited number of clinical trials for these pathologies. However, recent decades have seen **significant therapeutic advances**, thanks in particular to advances in genetics and biotechnology, and growing recognition of the importance of rare diseases in medical research. These advances have led to a better understanding of the mechanisms underlying some of these diseases, paving the way for innovative treatments such as **gene therapies**, **targeted therapies** and **orphan drugs**. However, the management of these diseases remains complex, marked by major challenges, particularly in terms of access to treatments and participation in clinical trials.

Therapeutic advances

Among the most notable advances, **gene therapy** stands out as a revolution in the treatment of certain rare diseases. This approach involves introducing, replacing or correcting a defective gene in a patient's cells, with the aim of treating or curing the disease at source. An emblematic example is the treatment of **spinal muscular atrophy** using innovative gene therapy. This neurodegenerative disease, which causes motor neuron degeneration and progressive muscle atrophy, has historically benefited from few effective treatments. The introduction of gene therapy has enabled some young patients to improve their life expectancy and quality of life, by stabilizing or slowing the progression of the disease. Although promising, this type of treatment remains costly and complex to administer, and is only accessible in specialized reference centers.

Another area of progress is the development of **orphan drugs**. These drugs are specifically designed to treat rare diseases, and are often the result of intensive biotechnology research. Due to the small number of patients involved, the development of these treatments is often unprofitable for pharmaceutical companies, which explains the need for incentives, such as subsidies and tax breaks, to encourage research in this field. Thanks to these efforts, a number of innovative treatments have been developed, notably for diseases such as **cystic fibrosis**, where drugs targeting the disease's specific genetic mutations have considerably improved patients' quality of life and survival.

Targeted therapies, which target specific abnormalities at cellular or molecular level, also represent a major advance in the treatment of rare cancers, such as **Ewing's sarcoma** or certain types of rare leukemia. These treatments make it possible to attack cancer cells directly while preserving healthy cells, thus reducing side effects and improving treatment efficacy. However, their development remains long and costly, and access to them may be limited by the availability of treatments in certain countries, or by their high cost.

The challenges of care

Despite these advances, treating rare diseases remains a **major challenge**. One of the main difficulties lies in **diagnosing** these diseases. Because of the rarity of the pathologies, it is not uncommon for patients to go through a long period of medical wandering before obtaining a precise diagnosis. This wandering, which can last for years, is a source of frustration and suffering for both patients and their families. What's more, many general practitioners and specialists are unfamiliar with these rare pathologies, which further delays access to appropriate care.

The **lack of available treatments** is another obstacle. Although progress has been made with gene therapies and orphan drugs, many rare diseases still have no curative treatment, and management remains essentially symptomatic. This means that patients are often faced with heavy treatments to manage symptoms, with no hope of a cure. For some patients, access to available treatments is also limited by their prohibitive cost. Innovative therapies, such as gene treatments, can cost hundreds of thousands of euros, and healthcare systems in some countries cannot always cover these expenses.

Another major challenge is **access to clinical trials**. Clinical trials play a crucial role in the development of new treatments for rare diseases, but participation in these trials is often difficult. Due to the rarity of the diseases, recruiting patients for trials can be time-consuming and complex. In addition, clinical trials are often conducted in specialized centers, which can require extensive travel for patients and their families. This geographical and logistical constraint can be a major barrier to participation, especially as rare disease patients are often in a fragile state of health, making travel difficult. Access to clinical trials can also be unequal in different parts of the world, further exacerbating inequalities in care.

Strict regulatory standards and lack of funding are also obstacles to setting up clinical trials for rare diseases. Pharmaceutical companies are sometimes reluctant to invest in costly trials for a limited market, despite existing incentives. In addition, clinical trials in rare diseases often require a personalized approach, with very small patient cohorts, which can complicate trial design and lengthen trial duration. Patients may have to wait a long time before trials become available, and eligibility criteria may exclude certain patients on the basis of their disease stage or other characteristics.

Solutions to improve care

In the face of these challenges, solutions are beginning to emerge. **European** and international **reference networks** for rare diseases, such as the **Centers of Reference for Rare Diseases**, play a crucial role in improving patient care. These centers bring together medical and scientific expertise in dedicated structures, offering patients access to multidisciplinary teams specialized in their disease. These networks also facilitate access to clinical trials and innovative treatments, while fostering collaborative research on an international scale.

Improved **neonatal screening** for certain rare diseases is also a major step forward. Thanks to early genetic testing, certain pathologies can now be detected at birth, enabling immediate and preventive treatment. This type of screening is already in place for diseases such as **cystic fibrosis** and certain **metabolic disorders**, and its expansion could significantly improve the prognosis of many other rare diseases.

Chapter 10

Nutrition and the importance of dietary care in hematology

The impact of hematological treatments on patients' nutritional status.
Treatment side effects (loss of appetite, mucositis, nausea) and their impact on nutrition.

The **side effects of treatments** for serious illnesses, particularly those associated with chemotherapy, radiotherapy and immunotherapy, can have a major impact on patients' nutritional status. Among the most common side effects are **loss of appetite**, **mucositis** (inflammation and ulceration of the mucous membranes of the mouth and digestive tract), and **nausea**. These symptoms, though often unavoidable, must be carefully managed, as they can lead to severe undernutrition, affecting the patient's ability to tolerate treatment and maintain strength.

Loss of appetite

Loss of appetite, or anorexia, is one of the most common side-effects of cancer treatments and other severe therapies. Chemotherapy and radiotherapy can alter the taste of food, provoke feelings of disgust or simply reduce the desire to eat due to the patient's general fatigue. Changes in metabolism, often induced by these treatments, can also play a role in loss of appetite. In some patients, even the smell or sight of food can provoke nausea, making eating extremely difficult.

The direct consequence of this loss of appetite is a reduction in caloric intake, which often leads to involuntary weight loss. The loss of energy and nutrients weakens the body, slowing tissue healing and reducing tolerance to treatments. To counteract this loss of appetite, it is important to adapt meals to the patient's tolerances, giving priority to calorie- and protein-rich foods, but in smaller, more frequent forms. Splitting meals into several smaller portions over the course of the day can help reduce food aversion while ensuring adequate nutritional intake.

It may also be useful to modify the texture of foods to suit the patient's preferences or the constraints imposed by other side effects, such as mucositis. **Oral nutritional supplements** can be prescribed to ensure adequate energy intake, notably in the form of beverages enriched in protein and calories, and containing essential vitamins and minerals. These solutions can compensate for reduced food intake, especially when the patient is unable to tolerate solid foods.

Mucositis

Mucositis, or inflammation of the mucous membranes of the mouth, throat and sometimes the entire digestive tract, is another common side effect, especially in patients undergoing chemotherapy or radiotherapy to the head and neck. Mucositis manifests itself as ulcerations, intense pain and difficulty swallowing, making eating extremely painful and sometimes impossible. These lesions can also encourage secondary infections, worsening the patient's general state of health.

The nutritional consequences of mucositis are significant. The inability to eat solid foods, and sometimes even liquids, leads to **rapid undernutrition** if appropriate measures are not taken. Patients often need a modified diet, with textures that are easier to swallow, such as purées, soups or liquid foods. It is essential to **protect the mucous membranes** by avoiding irritating foods, such as those that are acidic, spicy, salty or very hot, as these can aggravate lesions and accentuate pain. The use of antiseptic or anesthetic mouthwashes before meals can temporarily alleviate pain, making eating easier.

For patients suffering from severe mucositis, who can no longer swallow at all, more invasive solutions, such as **enteral** (gastric tube) or even **parenteral** (intravenous) **nutrition**, may be necessary to ensure adequate nutritional intake and avoid severe undernutrition. These approaches are reserved for cases where oral feeding becomes impossible, but they do help to maintain essential calorie and nutrient intake to support the patient throughout treatment.

Nausea and vomiting

Nausea and **vomiting**, often induced by chemotherapy or radiotherapy, also represent a major obstacle to normal eating. These symptoms can be constant or occur in waves, particularly after treatment sessions. **Repeated vomiting** not only leads to a loss of desire to eat, but can also cause **dehydration** and **electrolyte imbalance**, aggravating the patient's fatigue and weakness. Moreover, patients who vomit frequently may develop an aversion to certain foods that they associate with these episodes of unhappiness, further restricting their diet.

Nausea management relies mainly on the administration of **antiemetic drugs**, prescribed before and after treatment sessions. These drugs limit the intensity of nausea and vomiting, making it easier to eat. However, it is also important to adapt the diet to reduce the risk of triggering nausea. Meals should be **light, divided into small portions**, and composed of easily digestible foods such as starchy foods, cooked vegetables and lean proteins. Avoid fatty, fried, spicy or sweet foods, which can aggravate nausea. Eating cold or lukewarm foods, rather than hot ones, can also help limit feelings of disgust.

Hydration is a critical point in the management of nausea and vomiting, as repeated vomiting can lead to rapid dehydration. It is important to encourage the patient to drink small amounts of fluids regularly, especially electrolyte-rich beverages, to compensate for water and mineral losses. Light teas, clear broths or isotonic beverages can be helpful in maintaining a good level of hydration without overloading the stomach.

Overall impact on nutrition and quality of life

The **side effects** of treatment, whether loss of appetite, mucositis or nausea, have a major impact on patients' nutritional status. **Undernutrition**, which can set in rapidly if these side effects are not managed effectively, considerably weakens the body and can compromise the efficacy of ongoing treatments. A precarious nutritional state slows healing, reduces immune defenses, and can lead to greater susceptibility to infections, post-operative complications, and poorer tolerance of treatments.

It is therefore essential to adopt a proactive, **individualized** approach to managing these side effects. The role of **dieticians** and **nutritional support teams** is essential in adapting the diet to the specific needs of each patient, taking into account their symptoms and food preferences. Personalized nutritional strategies help avoid excessive weight loss and maintain a nutrient intake that supports recovery.

Specific dietary recommendations in hematology
Diets adapted to each situation: immunocompromised patients, transplant patients, end-of-life patients, etc.

Nutrition plays an essential role in the management of patients with serious illnesses, and diets must be adapted to the specific features of each clinical situation. Whether for **immunocompromised** patients, **transplant** patients, or those at the **end of life,** the main objective is to ensure adequate nutritional intake to support the body, improve quality of life, and prevent or limit health-related complications. These diets, while sharing certain common principles, must be adjusted to the specific needs of each patient, taking into account ongoing treatments and the constraints imposed by the disease.

Diet for immunocompromised patients

Immunocompromised patients, whether undergoing chemotherapy, leukemia or bone marrow transplants, are at increased risk of infection due to their weakened immune systems. In this context, diet must be strictly controlled to **minimize the risk of foodborne infections**, while maintaining sufficient nutritional intake to support healing and strengthen the body's defenses.

The diet recommended for immunocompromised patients is generally a **neutropenic diet**, aimed at avoiding the ingestion of potentially dangerous pathogens. This diet imposes strict rules of food hygiene, including the avoidance of raw or undercooked foods, which may contain bacteria, viruses or fungi that can cause infections. Raw fruit and vegetables must be carefully washed or peeled, and dairy products must be pasteurized. Meat, fish and eggs must be thoroughly cooked, and deli meats and soft cheeses are generally avoided, as they present a higher risk of contamination.

In addition to these precautions, it is essential to ensure adequate nutritional intake, as these patients, often weakened by treatment, can lose weight and suffer from malnutrition. Meals rich in **proteins**, **vitamins** and **minerals** are necessary to maintain muscle mass, support immune function and promote recovery. Nutritional supplements can be introduced if diet alone is insufficient to meet the patient's energy needs.

Diet for transplant patients

Transplant patients, whether bone marrow, liver, kidney or other organ transplants, require special attention to nutrition, not only to promote recovery after transplantation, but also to **prevent graft rejection** and **minimize the side effects** of immunosuppressive treatments. These treatments, which are essential to prevent rejection of the transplanted organ, weaken the patient's immune system, making him or her more vulnerable to infection, while also causing metabolic changes that can lead to nutritional imbalances.

In the first months following transplantation, a strict diet is often recommended. As with immunosuppressed patients, a **neutropenic diet** should be adopted to reduce the risk of foodborne infections. In addition, immunosuppressive drugs can cause side effects such as hyperglycemia, hypertension and fluid retention. The diet must therefore be adapted to take account of these issues, with restrictions on **sodium**, **fast sugars** and sometimes **saturated fats**, depending on the patient's state of health.

Transplant patients' diets must also be **rich in protein** to promote tissue healing and muscle regeneration after transplantation. Protein plays a key role in post-operative recovery, and lean protein sources such as poultry, fish or vegetable proteins are often recommended. **Antioxidant-rich foods**, such as cooked fruits and vegetables, can also be incorporated into the diet to support immune function without increasing the risk of infection. In the long term, regular monitoring of cholesterol, blood sugar and blood pressure levels is necessary, and diet must be adapted to prevent chronic complications.

Diet for patients at the end of life

Nutritional management of **patients at the end of life** differs from conventional approaches, in that the aim is no longer to prolong life, but to ensure **maximum comfort** and respect for the patient's needs and wishes. In these situations, it is not uncommon for the patient to experience a significant loss of appetite, linked to the disease itself, to the treatments, or to the general weakening of the organism. **Nausea**, **fatigue** and **pain** can also complicate eating.

In this context, the diet must be **flexible** and adapted to the patient's preferences and abilities. The idea is to **maintain as pleasant a diet as possible**, giving priority to foods that are easy to eat and that give the patient pleasure. Rather than insisting on calorie intake or strict nutritional requirements, the emphasis is on **frequent small portions** of foods that the patient enjoys, even if they are not always perfectly balanced. The pleasure of eating, however modest, can bring great emotional comfort.

In some cases, **artificial nutrition** (gastric tube or intravenous infusion) may be considered, but this is often discussed in the light of the patient's and family's wishes. When oral feeding becomes too difficult or painful, comfort and respect for the patient's wishes are paramount. It is also essential to avoid forced feeding, as this can cause unnecessary suffering, both physical and psychological.

Diet for cystic fibrosis patients

Cystic fibrosis patients have specific nutritional needs linked to malabsorption of nutrients, particularly fats. Due to the excessive production of thick mucus that obstructs the pancreatic ducts, these patients have difficulty digesting and properly absorbing fats and proteins, which can lead to severe malnutrition. Consequently, their diet must be **rich in calories** and **protein** to compensate for these losses.

Cystic fibrosis patients should also take **enzyme supplements** to improve fat and protein digestion. Meals should be rich in healthy fats, such as vegetable oils, oily fish or avocados, to provide a concentrated source of energy, while being accompanied by supplements of fat-soluble vitamins (A, D, E, K), which are often poorly absorbed due to the disease. We also recommend enriching meals with protein powders or food supplements to prevent weight loss.

The role of the caregiver in nutritional monitoring and support
How caregivers can identify risks of undernutrition, take part in prevention, and work with dieticians to adapt meals.

Caregivers play a crucial role in detecting the risk of undernutrition and implementing preventive measures, especially with fragile patients such as those suffering from chronic illnesses, cancer, or post-operative care. By working closely with patients on a day-to-day basis, caregivers are often the first to observe the subtle signs of reduced food intake, involuntary weight loss or deterioration in general condition, all of which are warning signs of undernutrition. Thanks to their role of observation and vigilance, they play an active role in preventing undernutrition, and work closely with dieticians and other members of the care team to adapt meals to the specific needs of each patient.

Identifying the risks of undernutrition

Early identification of the risk of undernutrition is essential to avoid a rapid deterioration in the patient's state of health. Through their regular contact with the patient, caregivers are particularly well placed to spot these early warning signs. Among the **key indicators** they can monitor are :

- **Visible weight loss**: the caregiver may observe rapid or progressive weight loss, often visible on the patient's face, arms or legs, which may indicate a reduction in food intake. It is important to note any change in morphology, however subtle, particularly in long-stay patients or those undergoing treatment for serious illnesses.

- **Decreased appetite**: if a patient shows less interest in food, eats smaller quantities than usual, or expresses a persistent lack of appetite, the caregiver should report this observation to the team. **Anorexia** may be due to the side-effects of treatment (chemotherapy, radiotherapy), pain, digestive problems or psychological disorders such as depression.

- **Difficulty chewing or swallowing**: patients suffering from **mucositis**, dry mouth or other swallowing disorders may have difficulty eating normally. The caregiver can spot these problems by observing the way the patient eats, or by being attentive to the patient's complaints about pain or discomfort during meals.

- **Excessive fatigue or weakness**: a drop in energy or intense fatigue, particularly if accompanied by muscle weakness, can be a sign of undernutrition. Caregivers must be vigilant if a patient finds it increasingly difficult to get up, walk or perform simple everyday tasks.

- **Skin changes and slow healing**: the skin may become drier, more fragile, or marked by wounds that are slow to heal in cases of malnutrition. The caregiver, in charge of hygiene and regular observation of the patient's body, is often the first to notice these signs.

- **Changes in behaviour or mood**: undernutrition can also affect a patient's mental and emotional state. **Increased irritability**, moments of confusion, or a tendency to isolate can be indirect indicators of inadequate nutrition.

Help prevent undernutrition

Once **signs of undernutrition** or potential risks have been identified, the caregiver plays an active role in prevention, adjusting certain aspects of care to encourage the patient to eat better, and promptly alerting the medical team if necessary. Here are a few actions he/she can take to prevent undernutrition:

- **Encourage patients to eat regularly**: the caregiver can propose split meals, distributed throughout the day in small portions, for patients who find it difficult to eat full meals. They can also monitor the snacks offered between meals to ensure that patients, particularly those at risk, are getting enough calories.

- **Ensuring comfort during meals**: it's important to make sure that the patient is comfortable when eating. Pain, breathing difficulties or an uncomfortable position can make eating difficult. The caregiver can adjust the patient's position, by raising the back of the bed or providing pillows to facilitate swallowing.

- **Encourage a pleasant environment**: meals should be taken in a calm, soothing environment. The caregiver can avoid distractions (such as television or outside noise) and create a pleasant atmosphere to encourage the patient to eat. They can also encourage the patient to eat in company, if possible, to make the moment more convivial and stimulating.

- **Adapting food texture**: some patients have difficulty chewing or swallowing. The caregiver can suggest or prepare foods that are easier to eat, such as purées, soups or soft foods. In the case of patients suffering from mucositis or swallowing disorders, these adaptations help limit pain and maintain adequate food intake.

- **Monitor hydration**: in addition to food, hydration is crucial, especially for elderly patients or those with swallowing disorders. The caregiver must ensure that the patient drinks regularly throughout the day, offering small quantities of water, broth or diluted juice if necessary.

Collaboration with dieticians

Collaboration with dieticians is a fundamental aspect of managing patients at risk of undernutrition. The caregiver, who is with the patient on a daily basis, plays a key role in passing on observations to the dieticians, so that they can adapt meals to the patient's specific needs. This collaboration is based on regular communication and the implementation of joint strategies to optimize nutritional intake.

- **Passing on accurate information**: when caregivers observe signs of undernutrition, they must promptly inform the dieticians. This includes information on food consumption (amount of food eaten, type of food rejected), the patient's food preferences, any difficulties encountered (chewing pain, digestive problems), as well as physical signs of undernutrition (weight loss, fatigue).

- **Adapting meals**: Based on the information provided, dieticians can adapt meals to better suit the patient's abilities and needs. This may include enriching meals with proteins, nutritional supplements or vitamins, adjusting textures, or modifying menus to take account of the patient's dietary preferences and tolerances. The caregiver may need to adjust the presentation of dishes, add condiments to enhance taste, or suggest easier-to-eat alternatives.

- **Follow-up**: Once the dietary recommendations have been implemented, the caregiver monitors the patient's reaction. He/she must ensure that the patient is eating better and that the adjustments made are well tolerated. If difficulties persist, it is essential to return to the dieticians to readjust the diet.

- **Nutritional education**: Caregivers can also play a role in educating patients and their families about nutrition-related issues. They can explain the importance of a healthy diet to support treatment, encourage the patient to try food supplements, or offer practical advice to make eating at home easier if necessary.

Chapter 11

Risk prevention and management in hematology

Infectious risks: prevention of nosocomial infections and asepsis management.
Rigorous hygiene practices to avoid infections.

Rigorous hygiene practices are essential to prevent infections, particularly in medical environments where patients are vulnerable, such as hematology, intensive care and transplant units. Immunocompromised patients, those undergoing chemotherapy, or those who have undergone major surgery, are particularly at risk of contracting infections that can have serious, even fatal, consequences. Nosocomial infections, i.e. those contracted in hospital, represent a real threat in these settings, and strict hygiene protocols are essential to minimize this risk.

As the patient's first point of contact on a daily basis, the nursing auxiliary plays a crucial role in the application of these **hygiene measures,** and must comply with rigorous practices to limit the risk of infection. These measures concern the personal hygiene of caregivers as much as that of patients, and the upkeep of the care environment.

Hand hygiene: the first line of defense

Hand disinfection is the cornerstone of infection prevention in any medical setting. The majority of nosocomial infections are transmitted by the hands, whether during direct patient care or through the handling of medical devices or contaminated surfaces. It is therefore imperative for caregivers to strictly follow hand hygiene protocols, whether by washing with soap and water or using hydroalcoholic solutions.

The **key moments** for hand disinfection are well defined and include:

- **Before and after any contact with a patient**.
- **Before performing aseptic care**, such as handling an infusion or dressing.

- **After contact with body fluids**, blood, secretions or excretions, even if gloves have been worn.
- **After touching the patient's environment**, including the bed, medical devices or any other object in the room.

Hands should be **washed with** care, rubbing each part of the hand for at least 30 seconds, including the back of the hands, the interdigital spaces and under the fingernails. If hands are not visibly dirty, rubbing with a hydroalcoholic solution is sufficient, provided it covers the entire surface of the hands and is applied until complete evaporation.

Wearing personal protective equipment (PPE)

The correct use of **personal protective equipment (PPE)** is essential to protect both caregivers and patients from cross-infection. PPE includes **gloves**, **gowns** or overcoats, **masks**, and sometimes **goggles** or **visors**, depending on the care provided.

- **Gloves** must be worn whenever in contact with body fluids, mucous membranes or wounds. It is crucial to change them between each patient, and even during care if moving from a contaminated area to a clean one, to avoid cross-contamination. After use, gloves should be removed in such a way as not to contaminate hands, and hands should be disinfected immediately after removal.

- **Gowns** or overcoats are used in high-risk departments, such as transplant or intensive care units, to protect caregivers' clothing from potential contaminants. They must be changed between each patient and removed before leaving the room to avoid transporting pathogens from one place to another.

- **Masks** are essential, especially to protect immunocompromised patients from infectious agents carried by caregivers. They must be worn when there is a risk of droplet transmission, such as during respiratory care or in the presence of patients with airborne diseases.

The mask must fit properly and must never be touched once in place.

Medical device hygiene and waste management

Medical devices used on patients, whether catheters, infusions or respiratory equipment, must be handled with the utmost care, as they are potential routes of entry for infections. The caregiver must follow sterilization and disinfection protocols for each device, ensuring that the equipment used is sterile or properly disinfected before each use.

Medical **waste management** is also a critical factor in preventing the spread of infectious agents. Infectious risk waste (syringes, used dressings, etc.) must be disposed of in specific, watertight and secure containers, to avoid any risk of accidental contamination. These containers must be emptied regularly, in accordance with current protocols, and handled with gloves to limit the risk of exposure.

Hygiene of surfaces and care environments

Maintaining a clean and disinfected environment is essential to limit the proliferation of pathogens in areas where patients are cared for. Caregivers must ensure that **frequent contact surfaces** (door handles, handrails, light switches, bedside tables) are regularly cleaned and disinfected with suitable products.

Patient rooms, especially those of immunocompromised or transplant patients, must be cleaned according to **strict protocols**. Bed linen and clothing must be changed regularly, and all reusable equipment (such as bedpans and toiletries) must be thoroughly disinfected between uses.

Additional precautions for patients in isolation

Patients in isolation (such as immunocompromised patients or those with contagious infections) require extra precautions to prevent the transmission of infections. For these patients, caregivers must follow reinforced protocols, which include not only the wearing of PPE, but also strict rules for entering and leaving the room.

For immunocompromised patients, particularly those who have undergone transplantation, **protective isolation** measures are put in place to prevent exposure to outside germs. This includes the systematic wearing of gowns, gloves and masks by all caregivers and visitors, as well as strict rules on hand and surface disinfection before any contact with the patient.

Patient and family education

Finally, the caregiver also plays a key role in **educating patients and their families** about hygiene. They can explain the rules to be followed to prevent infection, such as the importance of hand washing, the use of masks in certain contexts, or the precautions to be taken when handling medical devices in the home. This education is essential to ensure that patients and their families are actively involved in infection prevention, both in hospital and when they return home.

Preventing movement and posture-related risks in bedridden patients
The importance of passive mobilization, pressure sore and thrombosis prevention.

Passive mobilization, as well as the **prevention of pressure sores** and **thrombosis**, is of paramount importance in the care of bedridden patients or those with reduced mobility. These patients, often recovering from surgery or suffering from chronic or neurological illnesses, are particularly at risk of serious complications associated with prolonged immobility. As a key player in day-to-day care, the nursing auxiliary plays a central role in implementing passive mobilization techniques and preventing complications such as bedsores and venous thrombosis, thereby helping to improve patient comfort, quality of life and safety.

The importance of passive mobilization

Passive mobilization involves moving the patient's joints and limbs without effort. This technique is often used with immobilized, comatose or paralyzed patients who are unable to move on their own. Although the patient is passive, this mobilization is essential to maintain joint flexibility, prevent muscle stiffness and avoid complications associated with immobility.

One of the main aims of passive mobilization is to **prevent joint ankylosis**, i.e. the loss of joint mobility due to inactivity. When a patient remains immobile for long periods, muscles and joints can stiffen, making movement painful and even leading to permanent loss of joint function. Passive mobilization helps to maintain joint flexibility and preserve range of motion. It also stimulates blood circulation in the limbs, helping to prevent complications such as thrombosis.

Passive mobilization is also beneficial in **preventing respiratory complications**. In bedridden patients, breathing is often shallower, which can encourage the accumulation of secretions in the lungs, leading to respiratory infections such as pneumonia. By mobilizing the limbs and encouraging regular position changes, the caregiver helps to **improve respiratory capacity** by promoting better thoracic expansion.

Pressure sore prevention

Pressure sores, or pressure ulcers, are skin lesions that form when blood circulation is compromised due to prolonged pressure on certain parts of the body. They frequently occur in bedridden patients or those with reduced mobility, particularly in bony areas such as the heels, sacrum, hips and elbows. The prevention of pressure sores is a priority in the care of immobilized patients, as these lesions can lead to intense pain, serious infections and a general deterioration in health.

One of the most effective ways of preventing pressure sores is to **regularly change the patient's position** to avoid prolonged pressure on the same areas of the body. Caregivers should ensure that they **change position** every two hours or so, making sure that sensitive areas are relieved of pressure. The use of suitable equipment, such as air mattresses or anti-bedsore cushions, also helps to reduce pressure on at-risk areas and promote a more even distribution of body weight.

In addition to position changes, **skin hygiene** is essential to prevent pressure sores. The skin of immobilized patients is often more fragile and more prone to irritation. The caregiver must therefore ensure that the skin is clean and well moisturized, and avoid excessive rubbing that could aggravate skin irritation. In the event of early signs of pressure sores, such as persistent redness, it's crucial to act quickly by alerting the nursing team so that additional preventive measures can be put in place, such as the use of specific dressings or skin protectors.

Preventing venous thrombosis

Venous thrombosis, or blood clots, is another major complication of immobilized patients. Prolonged immobility slows blood flow, particularly in the lower limbs, increasing the risk of clot formation in the deep veins of the legs (deep vein thrombosis, or DVT). If a clot breaks loose, it can migrate to the lungs and cause a pulmonary embolism, a potentially fatal medical emergency. It is therefore imperative to prevent the formation of these clots in at-risk patients.

Passive mobilization helps prevent thrombosis by stimulating blood circulation. Regular movement of the lower limbs, even by the caregiver, helps to activate venous circulation and reduce blood stasis in the leg veins. Caregivers can also encourage patients capable of partial movement to perform simple exercises, such as flexing and extending the feet and legs, to promote venous return.

The use of **elastic restraints**, such as compression stockings or bandages, is another important preventive measure. These devices help maintain even pressure on the legs and improve blood circulation, particularly in bedridden or post-operative patients. The caregiver plays a key role in the correct application of these devices, and must ensure that compression stockings fit snugly, without creating creases or extra pressure points.

Finally, **clinical monitoring** for signs of venous thrombosis is essential. Caregivers must be alert to warning signs, such as sudden swelling of a leg, pain or unusual redness, and report any abnormalities immediately. Early attention can prevent serious complications and ensure prompt treatment, often with anticoagulants.

Collaboration and vigilance in preventing complications

Preventing pressure sores and **thrombosis** requires a **proactive approach** and constant monitoring. Because of their proximity to the patient, caregivers are often on the front line in identifying early signs of complications and implementing preventive measures. They work closely with nurses and doctors to adapt care to the patient's condition, and adjust interventions where necessary.

This vigilance also extends to **educating patients and their families**. In some cases, such as during convalescence at home, the caregiver can explain to relatives how to carry out position changes, how to monitor the skin, and how to help mobilize limbs, in order to extend preventive care outside the hospital setting.

Safety protocols for administering treatments (chemotherapy, transfusions, etc.).
The importance of double-checking and rigor in handling high-risk treatments.

Double-checking and **rigorous** handling of **high-risk treatments** are fundamental pillars in guaranteeing **patient safety** and avoiding errors that could have serious or even fatal consequences. These treatments, which include drugs such as chemotherapy, anticoagulants, opioids and insulin, require special attention at every stage of preparation and administration. Working closely with nurses and pharmacists, caregivers must apply strict verification and control protocols, to ensure that treatments are given correctly, to the right patient, at the right dose and at the right time.

Handling high-risk treatments: a shared responsibility

High-risk treatments are those which, if administered incorrectly, can lead to severe side effects or potentially fatal complications for the patient. Responsibility for their administration rests with the entire health-care team, but each health-care professional involved in the process plays a specific role. Although not always directly responsible for drug administration, the caregiver is often involved in the **preparation** and **monitoring** of the patient, giving him or her a crucial role in the safety of the process.

For example, when preparing infusions or handling medical devices such as infusion pumps, caregivers must follow **precise, standardized protocols**. These protocols are designed to minimize errors by introducing verification steps at each phase of the process, from checking the prescription to administering the treatment.

The importance of double-checking

Double-checking is an essential practice when it comes to high-risk drugs. It involves two members of the healthcare team, usually a nurse and an orderly, jointly checking several aspects of the treatment before it is administered. This collaborative process reduces human error by bringing together two professional perspectives.

Key elements to be verified as part of a double check include :

- **The right drug**: Ensuring that the medication prepared is the one prescribed. This involves checking the **exact name of** the drug, taking into account any similarities between certain drug names that could lead to confusion.
- **The right dose**: It's vital to ensure that the **dose prescribed** corresponds to the dose actually administered,

especially in the case of powerful drugs such as chemotherapy or anticoagulants, where even a small error in dosage can have serious consequences.

- **Route of administration**: Each drug must be administered by the **appropriate route** (intravenous, oral, subcutaneous, etc.). Confusing routes of administration can lead to inadequate absorption or toxic effects.
- **The right patient**: The patient's identity must be systematically verified before treatment is administered, using at least two identifiers, such as the identification bracelet and date of birth or file number. This verification is all the more important in hospital environments where several patients receive similar treatments.
- **The right time**: Certain high-risk treatments need to be administered at specific times, and a **rigorous timetable** is essential to respect hourly doses, avoid overdosing or minimize drug interactions.

This cross-checking between two professionals offers an **additional guarantee of safety**, as it reduces the risk of error due to distraction, fatigue or misreading of the prescription.

Rigorous adherence to protocols

In addition to double-checking, **rigorous** adherence to protocols is essential to ensure patient safety. Every step, from preparation to post-administration monitoring, must be scrupulously followed, with no shortcuts or improvisations. The handling of **high-risk drugs** requires specific precautions to ensure that every gesture is carried out with precision.

An important aspect of this rigor concerns the **sterile preparation** of injectable drugs. Chemotherapies, for example, must be prepared under rigorous aseptic conditions to avoid any contamination that could endanger the patient, particularly when treating immunocompromised patients. Nurses involved in the preparation of devices for administration (such as infusion preparation) must adhere strictly to hygiene and sterilization standards.

Traceability of administered medication is another key element. Each drug administered must be recorded in the patient's file, indicating the dose, the time and the professional who administered it. This traceability is crucial to **avoid errors** when changing shifts, and enables precise monitoring of treatment progress, especially when several high-risk drugs are administered in parallel.

Post-administration monitoring: an essential role

Once treatments have been administered, **close monitoring of** patients is necessary, particularly for high-risk treatments that can lead to serious side effects. The caregiver plays an essential role in this ongoing monitoring, observing the patient's clinical signs that could indicate an adverse reaction, such as sudden pain, nausea, breathing difficulties, or changes in consciousness.

The caregiver's vigilance is all the more crucial in the first few hours following the administration of drugs such as anticoagulants or chemotherapy, as these treatments can lead to acute complications such as excessive bleeding or allergic reactions. In the event of any anomaly, the caregiver must immediately alert the nurse or doctor, so that corrective action can be taken without delay.

Team collaboration and communication

Fluid communication within the healthcare team is also essential to ensure the safety of high-risk treatments. Working closely with nurses, pharmacists and doctors, the caregiver must ensure that all necessary information concerning the patient and his or her treatment is shared. This communication is all the more crucial during **team transmissions**, where any omission or confusion in the transmission of information can lead to treatment errors.

It's also important for the caregiver to take an active part in **multidisciplinary meetings** or informal exchanges with the medical team, to discuss any necessary adjustments to treatments based on the patient's condition. By adopting a proactive and rigorous attitude, the caregiver not only helps to ensure the safe administration of treatments, but also anticipates and prevents possible complications.

Chapter 12

Occupational health for hematology nurses

Physical risks associated with repetitive tasks and heavy loads
MSD prevention, adapted gestures and postures, use of handling equipment.

Preventing musculoskeletal disorders (MSDs) is a priority for healthcare professionals, especially for care assistants, whose daily tasks include **carrying heavy loads, mobilizing patients and** numerous repetitive manipulations. MSDs mainly affect muscles, tendons and joints, causing chronic pain that can lead to an inability to work. To prevent these risks, it is essential to adopt **appropriate gestures and postures**, and to use **handling equipment** correctly.

Understanding MSDs and their impact

MSDs are disorders that occur as a result of repeated stress, poor posture or excessive strain on the body, mainly in the back, shoulders, neck, wrists and knees. These conditions are common among care assistants, who are constantly straining their muscles and joints as they help patients get up, move around, or perform hygiene tasks. MSDs can manifest themselves as diffuse pain, joint stiffness, loss of strength or mobility, and, in the most serious cases, lead to prolonged work stoppages.

The prevention of MSDs is therefore based on two main principles: **the adoption of correct postures and gestures** during handling, and the use of suitable **handling equipment** to reduce physical effort. This not only preserves the health of caregivers, but also improves the quality of care provided to patients, by guaranteeing their safety during movements and transfers.

Appropriate gestures and postures

The adoption of **appropriate gestures and postures** is essential to prevent MSDs. These are techniques designed to reduce the

136

mechanical stress on the body during repetitive movements or the handling of loads, by optimizing the use of muscles and joints.

1. **Bend the knees, not the back**: When it comes to lifting a patient or a heavy object, it's crucial to **bend the knees** rather than bend forward and arch the back. This posture uses the leg muscles, which are more powerful, rather than the spine. It's important to keep the back straight throughout the movement to avoid straining the lumbar vertebrae.

2. **Keep the load close to the body**: When transporting or moving a patient or object, it is advisable to **keep the load as close to the body as possible**. This reduces the lever arm and therefore the strain on the back muscles. The further the load is from the body, the greater the pressure on the spine, increasing the risk of injury.

3. **Anticipate movements**: Before moving a patient, it's essential to **prepare the movement** and ensure that all the necessary equipment is at hand. The space must be clear, and the caregiver must be in a stable posture, with feet slightly apart, to ensure good balance. This helps avoid sudden movements or imbalances, which are often the cause of injury.

4. **Teamwork**: For particularly heavy tasks, such as transferring a patient from a bed to a chair, we recommend **working** in **pairs** or groups. Sharing the load considerably reduces the physical effort for each caregiver and ensures better control of movement. Prior coordination between team members is necessary to synchronize actions and avoid uncoordinated movements.

5. **Alternate postures and avoid prolonged static positions**: Prolonged immobility in an uncomfortable position can also cause RSI. It is therefore important to **alternate postures**, to avoid standing or sitting in the

same position for too long, and to take breaks to relax and stretch muscles.

Use of handling equipment

The use of suitable **handling equipment** is essential to reduce the physical load on caregivers and to guarantee patient safety. This equipment is designed to assist caregivers in **transferring** and **mobilizing patients**, while minimizing muscular effort and the risk of injury.

1. **Patient lift**: This equipment is particularly useful for transferring patients with very limited mobility. The **lift**, also known as a **patient lift**, enables the patient to be lifted and moved in complete safety, without the caregiver having to make an intense physical effort. A thorough understanding of the lift's operation is essential for its safe and optimal use. The caregiver must ensure that the sling is correctly positioned on the patient before starting the transfer.

2. **Glide sheets and transfer boards**: **Glide sheets** are devices that facilitate the movement of patients in bed, or their transfer from a bed to a chair, for example. Thanks to their low-friction properties, these sheets **reduce the effort** required to slide the patient, thus limiting strain on the caregiver's shoulders and back. **Transfer boards** are also useful for transferring patients from one surface to another, without having to lift them completely.

3. **Transfer belts**: **Transfer belts** are ergonomic devices that the caregiver can fasten around the patient's waist to assist movement. They help guide and support the patient, while providing a better grip for the caregiver, reducing the risk of slipping or falling.

4. **Adjustable wheelchairs and healthcare beds**: The use of **adjustable wheelchairs** and **medical beds** enables the

patient's position to be adapted to the task in hand, thus reducing the effort required of caregivers. Height-adjustable beds, for example, allow the working height to be adjusted to avoid excessive bending or stooping.

Raising awareness and continuing education

The **prevention of MSDs** also relies on **ongoing training** and **regular awareness-raising** among caregivers of the appropriate gestures and postures. **Practical workshops** on ergonomics in the workplace and the correct use of handling equipment help them acquire the skills they need to protect their bodies. It's vital that every caregiver understands the importance of these practices in preserving their long-term health.

Establishing a **culture of prevention** within healthcare establishments, where caregivers are encouraged to systematically use available handling equipment and adopt the right postures, is an essential lever for reducing the incidence of MSDs. **Communication** between colleagues is also key: caregivers must be encouraged to ask for help when they feel that a task may exceed their physical capabilities.

Managing stress and fatigue on a daily basis
Strategies to prevent physical and mental exhaustion: organization of work time, breaks, relaxation.

Preventing **physical and mental burnout** is a crucial issue for care assistants, whose profession demands not only a heavy physical workload, but also a high level of emotional involvement. The risk of **burnout** is particularly high in this sector, due to the repetitive and demanding nature of the tasks, as well as the emotional demands of caring for patients who are often in great distress. To prevent burnout, it is essential to implement **effective strategies** based on **optimal organization of working hours**, the importance of **regular breaks**, and the integration of **relaxation** techniques into daily life.

Organization of working hours

Well thought-out organization of working hours is essential to avoid overload and enable efficient management of tasks, without accumulating unnecessary stress. In often demanding environments, such as hospitals or retirement homes, caregivers have to juggle physical care, patient assistance, equipment management and team coordination. The right balance between these tasks **optimizes time** and reduces fatigue.

1. **Prioritizing tasks**: It's essential to learn to **prioritize tasks** according to their urgency and importance. Care requiring immediate attention, such as managing critical patients, should be given priority, while administrative or secondary tasks can be scheduled for less busy times. This approach allows you to stay focused on the most crucial aspects of the job without being overwhelmed by less urgent details.

2. **Balance between physical and mental tasks**: It's important to alternate between tasks that place heavy demands on the body, such as mobilizing or transferring patients, and those that are less physically demanding, such as case management or monitoring. This alternation helps limit physical fatigue while ensuring continuity in patient care.

3. **Planning break times**: Good organization of working hours also includes planning **regular breaks**. These moments of respite, well distributed throughout the day, allow you to recharge your batteries and avoid the accumulation of fatigue. For these breaks to be effective, they must be taken at the right time, before the caregiver feels exhausted. Respecting these breaks is essential, and

they should be seen not as a luxury, but as a necessity for maintaining a high level of alertness and efficiency.

The importance of regular breaks

Regular breaks play a key role in preventing burnout, both physical and mental. Working continuously without breaks exhausts the body's resources, leading to a drop in concentration, an increase in errors and a deterioration in the quality of care. **Short but frequent breaks** enable you to relax, release accumulated physical tension and refocus your mind.

1. **Physical break**: A **physical break** consists in interrupting activities that put a strain on muscles and joints, especially tasks requiring intense physical effort. This **releases muscular tension** and reduces the risk of musculoskeletal disorders (MSDs). During this break, we recommend gentle stretching exercises to relieve the most stressed areas of the body, such as shoulders, back or legs. Muscle relaxation is essential to avoid physical overload, which in the long term can lead to chronic pain.

2. **Mental break**: The aim of a **mental break** is to temporarily disconnect from stress and responsibilities. Working non-stop on emotionally or cognitively demanding tasks, such as caring for patients at the end of life, can quickly exhaust mental resources. During a mental break, the aim is to refocus on oneself, avoiding thoughts of upcoming tasks. Simple techniques, such as closing your eyes, breathing deeply or focusing on something positive, can help to calm the mind and release accumulated pressure.

3. **Microbreaks**: In addition to planned breaks, **microbreaks** are also very beneficial. These are short interruptions lasting just a few minutes that allow you to stand up, take a walk, or simply breathe deeply. These moments are particularly useful for restoring attention and

concentration, especially on busy days. Even a few moments of disconnection can be enough to reduce stress and recharge the batteries.

Integrating relaxation into everyday life

Relaxation is another essential component in preventing physical and mental exhaustion. Incorporating relaxation techniques into the day not only helps manage stress, but also promotes a general state of well-being, essential for maintaining a good quality of life at work.

1. **Breathing exercises**: **Deep breathing exercises** are one of the simplest and most effective ways to relax quickly. Taking a few minutes to concentrate on slow, deep breathing helps to reduce the heart rate and calm the mind. Diaphragmatic breathing, in which you breathe deeply, inflating the belly on the inhalation and relaxing it on the exhalation, helps to release accumulated tension and reduce anxiety.

2. **Meditation and mindfulness**: **Mindfulness meditation** is increasingly recognized for its stress management benefits. It involves paying attention to the present moment, without judgment, by concentrating on body sensations, breathing or surrounding sounds. Practicing mindfulness for even a few minutes during the day enables you to step back from stressful situations and return to your tasks with a calmer, more centered mind.

3. **Progressive muscle relaxation**: The **progressive muscle relaxation** technique is particularly useful for releasing physical tension accumulated over the course of the day. It involves progressively contracting and then releasing each muscle group, starting with the feet and working up to the head. This process helps you to become aware of areas of tension and effectively relax them, offering the body a moment's respite.

Long-term strategies to prevent burnout

Preventing burnout also requires **long-term strategies** aimed at achieving a lasting balance between work and rest. Among these strategies, the importance of **restful sleep** should not be underestimated. Accumulated sleep deprivation considerably increases the risk of chronic fatigue and burnout. Caregivers, who are often required to work irregular hours, need to adopt rigorous sleep hygiene, with regular schedules and an environment conducive to rest (dark, quiet room, pleasant temperature).

What's more, it's essential to **balance work and personal life**. Making time for pleasurable activities outside work, such as hobbies, family time or physical activity, is crucial to maintaining emotional balance. Regular light exercise, such as walking, yoga or swimming, reduces stress while strengthening the body.

Finally, not hesitating to **ask for help** or express your feelings is a key element in preventing burnout. It's important to have moments of exchange with colleagues or superiors to discuss the difficulties encountered, as unshared emotional overload can quickly lead to a state of intense mental fatigue. Support among colleagues strengthens team cohesion and provides a space to vent tensions.

The importance of work-life balance
How to maintain a healthy work-life balance in an emotionally and physically demanding work environment.

Maintaining a **healthy work-life balance** in a profession as emotionally and physically demanding as nursing is a real challenge. Caregivers are often confronted with stressful situations, heavy responsibilities and an intense emotional charge linked to accompanying suffering patients. This personal investment can sometimes encroach on private life, creating an imbalance which, in the long term, can lead to exhaustion, chronic stress and even **burnout**. However, with thoughtful strategies, it is possible to preserve this balance, ensuring both **mental health** and **personal satisfaction**.

Define clear boundaries between work and private life

The first step in maintaining a healthy balance is to **define clear boundaries** between work and private life. It's essential to **keep the two spheres separate**, to avoid work-related stress spilling over into personal life, and vice versa.

1. **Avoid bringing work home**: While it can be difficult to disconnect emotionally from difficult situations at work, it's crucial not to bring this burden home. This means, as far as possible, not mentally prolonging work concerns beyond the end of the day. Caregivers can give themselves a moment to decompress on leaving hospital, for example by practicing a few breathing exercises or listening to relaxing music, to mark the transition between work and home.

2. **Set reasonable working hours**: Irregular working hours or frequent overtime can quickly encroach on private life and physical recuperation. It's important to respect, as far as possible, a work rhythm that allows you to preserve time for yourself, family or leisure. Knowing how to say no to excessive demands, or limit overtime, is essential to avoid overwork and protect personal balance.

3. **Set up end-of-day rituals**: Another effective way of separating work and private life is to set up **end-of-day rituals**, which symbolically mark the end of the working day. This can include a relaxing walk, light physical activity, or a quiet moment for yourself, such as reading or meditation. These rituals allow you to refocus on your

personal needs and leave behind the stress accumulated at work.

Preserving time for yourself and your loved ones

To maintain a healthy balance, it's essential to **preserve time for yourself** and your loved ones, even when your workload is heavy. Personal relationships and moments of relaxation are sources of resourcefulness and comfort, essential to staying fulfilled, both personally and professionally.

1. **Make time for family and friends**: Interactions with loved ones play a key role in emotional support. It's important to schedule regular time with family or friends, to chat, share social moments and disconnect from work-related stress. Even short outings or simple activities such as a family dinner or a walk can have a beneficial effect on morale and help maintain balanced relationships.

2. **Make time for personal hobbies**: Caregivers must also take care to devote time to their own **hobbies** and passions. Whether it's sport, reading, music, or any other activity that brings pleasure and relaxation, these moments are essential to **recharge one's batteries** and regain psychological balance. By regularly integrating activities that bring happiness, it becomes easier to cope with the emotional demands of work.

3. **Physical and relaxation activities**: Physical exercise is an excellent way to release accumulated tension and relax mentally. Activities such as walking, running, swimming or yoga help to regulate stress while improving physical condition. **Relaxation techniques**, such as meditation or breathing exercises, are also powerful tools for regaining serenity and calming the mind after a hard day's work.

Managing work-related stress and emotions

In a demanding working environment, where patient suffering can be difficult to cope with, it's crucial to learn how to **manage stress** and **emotions** in a healthy way, so as not to let them take over your personal life.

1. **Talking about your emotions**: It's important to **share your feelings** with colleagues, friends and family. Communication helps to verbalize difficulties, find support and put stressful situations into perspective. Caregivers should not hesitate to talk to other members of the care team who are going through similar experiences, to share tips or simply for mutual support.

2. **Ask for help when you need it**: In cases of emotional overload or chronic stress, it's crucial not to hesitate to **ask for help**. This can involve consultations with a psychologist or stress counsellor, who can offer practical tools to better manage work-related emotions. Participating in **discussion groups** or **support groups** for caregivers can also be beneficial, enabling you to share your experience with other professionals facing the same challenges.

3. **Learning to let go**: It is essential to develop the ability to **let go** of situations that are beyond personal control. Caregivers are often confronted with difficult situations, such as suffering or death, which can be heavy to bear. Learning to accept that certain situations cannot be changed, and that we do our best in each circumstance, helps to reduce the weight of negative emotions.

Adapt expectations and remain flexible

Another key to maintaining a healthy life-work balance is to **readjust expectations** and adopt a flexible approach to the unexpected.

146

1. **Don't aim for perfection**: Trying to achieve everything, whether at work or at home, can quickly lead to exhaustion. It's important to accept that we can't always control everything, and that **perfection isn't attainable** in every aspect of life. Accepting one's limits and indulging oneself can help reduce pressure and avoid unnecessary stress.

2. **Staying flexible in the face of the unexpected**: In professions like nursing, it's not uncommon to have to deal with the unexpected, whether it's emergencies at work or unexpected personal obligations. It's essential to **remain flexible** and accept that certain situations require adjustments. This makes it easier to adapt to constraints without feeling frustrated or guilty.

Conclusion

The vocation of hematology caregiver

A reminder of the skills, human qualities and medical knowledge needed to excel in this department. The conclusion could also address the importance of commitment and passion for this profession, and the hope it offers patients.

To excel as an orderly in **hematology**, or in any other demanding medical department, it's essential to possess a diverse set of **technical skills**, **human qualities** and **medical knowledge**. This role is essential to accompany patients through what are often difficult times, and to provide day-to-day support to the care team, thereby contributing to the continuous improvement of care quality. Here's a reminder of the key elements that make the difference in this profession, on both technical and human levels.

Technical skills and medical knowledge

1. **Technical skills**: Caregivers must be able to perform basic care tasks with precision and rigor, such as taking vital signs (blood pressure, temperature, heart rate), assisting with toileting, hygiene and comfort care, as well as **preventive actions** such as mobilizing patients and preventing bedsores. In departments such as haematology, where patients may be immunocompromised or seriously ill, this care requires special attention to avoid the risk of infection or complications.

2. **Knowledge of specific pathologies**: Caregivers must also have a good understanding of the **main pathologies** treated in this type of department, such as leukemia, lymphoma or myeloma. Understanding the effects of treatments (chemotherapy, immunotherapy, radiotherapy) and the specific care they require is essential to responding appropriately to patients' needs. Managing side effects, such as nausea, mucositis or extreme fatigue, is an integral part of daily care.

3. **Use of medical equipment**: Caregivers must know how to handle **medical devices** safely, such as medical beds,

infusion pumps, monitoring devices or patient handling equipment (patient lifts, sliding sheets). Mastery of this equipment is crucial to guaranteeing safe care and minimizing risks for both patient and caregiver.

4. **Monitoring and observation**: An indispensable skill is the ability to **observe** patients **closely**, and quickly report any signs of deterioration or complication. Caregivers are often the first to notice subtle changes in a patient's condition, such as fever, increased weakness, or signs of infection or bleeding. Prompt communication with the nursing or medical team ensures fast, efficient care.

Essential human qualities

1. **Empathy and caring**: One of the foundations of the nursing profession is **empathy**, the ability to understand and feel what the patient is going through. When dealing with seriously ill, often suffering and vulnerable patients, active listening and benevolence are essential to create a climate of trust and comfort. These qualities also enable us to better support families, who are often worried and helpless when faced with their loved one's illness.

2. **Patience and calm**: **Patience** is an essential quality, as working with seriously ill patients can be long and demanding. Hematology patients can be tired, in pain, and sometimes frustrated by the slow progress or isolation of their treatment. It's crucial to maintain a calm, soothing attitude, even in tense moments, to help patients feel supported.

3. **Adaptability**: Hospital care, particularly in hematology, can be unpredictable. Caregivers must be able **to adapt quickly** to changing situations, whether a medical emergency, a change in treatment, or a rapid evolution in a patient's state of health. This flexibility enables them to

deal with the unforeseen with responsiveness and professionalism.

4. **Emotional resilience**: Working in hematology can be emotionally challenging. Caregivers are often confronted with suffering, chronic illness, and sometimes death. **Emotional resilience** is therefore crucial to staying engaged in your work while preserving your own mental well-being. Knowing how to step back, share your emotions with colleagues and resort to psychological support mechanisms is essential for coping with difficulties without burning out.

5. **Team spirit and communication**: Teamwork is at the heart of the nursing profession. Effective collaboration with nurses, doctors, physiotherapists and other healthcare professionals is essential to ensure complete patient care. **Good communication** is essential to pass on relevant information about the patient's condition, the care provided and any additional needs.

The importance of commitment and passion

Over and above technical skills and human qualities, what really makes the difference in the nursing auxiliary profession is **commitment** and **passion** for the role. Working in hematology, or in other demanding departments, demands a high level of personal commitment. Every day, caregivers provide not only physical care, but also **moral support** and **hope** to patients going through what are often difficult ordeals.

Commitment to this profession means accompanying patients in their daily struggles, listening to them, responding to their sometimes invisible needs, and offering comfort in moments of distress. Passion for the job is evident in the small gestures, the discreet attentions, and the deep satisfaction of knowing that we are helping to improve patients' quality of life, even in the most difficult situations.

Conclusion: A job that brings hope

Being an orderly, especially in a department as demanding as hematology, is much more than just a job. It's a deep commitment to humanity and an essential role in the care chain. **Passion** and **dedication** are at the heart of this profession, which demands not only medical skills, but also an ability to **sustain hope** in moments of great vulnerability.

For patients, contact with a caring, attentive and competent caregiver often represents a source of hope, a glimmer of comfort in a care journey that can sometimes be fraught with obstacles. By contributing their expertise and humanity, caregivers play an active part in this hope, in this **fight for life**, and help to transform the experience of patients and their families, even in the darkest moments.

In this way, the caregiver's commitment and passion are the pillars that not only underpin the quality of care, but also provide each patient with the hope, comfort and dignity they so desperately need.